LIVING CREATIVELY WITH CHRONIC ILLNESS

Developing Skills for Transcending The Loss, Pain and Frustration

LIVING CREATIVELY WITH CHRONIC ILLNESS

Developing Skills for Transcending The Loss, Pain and
Frustration

By

Eugenie G. Wheeler and Joyce Dace-Lombard

Pathfinder Publishing
458 Dorothy Ave.
Ventura, CA 93003
1989

LIVING CREATIVELY WITH CHRONIC ILLNESS
Developing Skills for Transcending The Loss,
Pain and Frustration

By

Eugenie G. Wheeler and Joyce Dace-Lombard

Edited by Ingrid Scott & Eugene D. Wheeler

Published By:
Pathfinder Publishing
458 Dorothy Avenue
Ventura, CA 93003
(805) 642-9278

Library of Congress Cataloging-in-Publication Data

Wheeler, Eugenie G., 1918-
   Living creatively with chronic illness.

   Bibliography: p.
   Includes index.
   1. Chronically ill--Rehabilitation. 2. Chronic
diseases--Psychological aspects. 3. Adjustment (Psy-
chology) I. Dace-Lombard, Joyce, 1935-   .
II. Title.
RC108.W43 1989   155.9'16   89-9250
ISBN 0-934793-17-4

DEDICATION

This Book is Dedicated to
people who cope with chronic illness
and inspire our lives with their creative living.

ACKNOWLEDGEMENTS

We appreciate most of all the input from the chronically ill people who so openly and generously shared their experiences, their feelings and their knowledge toward helping to make this book useful to others. As you meet them in the following chapters you will understand how moved we have been, and how deeply we appreciate their contributions.

We especially want to acknowledge the role of our publisher whose assistance went way beyond extensive editing and publishing. Without his encouragement, foresight and expertise this book would not have been written.

Ingrid Scott did a masterful job of editing which called upon her skills in conflict resolution as well as her considerable literary talents.

We appreciate Dr. Robert Gonzales' comprehensive review of the manuscript for medical accuracy.

A special thanks to those people profiled who helped with clarification in chapters that make reference to their coping skills. We are also indebted to Elsa Campbell for lending us her thesis, "Healing the Trauma of Diabetic Vision Loss."

We thank the numerous readers who were willing to give their time to reviewing the manuscript in whole or in part and to giving us their perceptive reactions and suggestions for improving it. Among them are Margaret P. Johnson, Ph.D., Psychologist and Jungian Analyst; Pickens Halt, M.S., MFCC, Hospice Bereavement Coordinator; Dr. Julie Kuehnel, Chair of the Psychology

Department, California Lutheran University; Jeanne Lindsay, Publisher, Morning Glory Press; Dinah Hamilton, LCSW, Director, Simi Counseling Center; Marsha and Burt Danet, Publishers and Editors, "Health Examiner;" Brett St. Giles, artist; and Lou Hartney, editor.

In addition, the "Book-Length Non-Fiction" group of the Ventura Writers' Club was a source of continuing support and competent critiquing for which we are also grateful.

Some students' input was also valuable, notably Linda Kapigian's paper on the impact of chronic illness on marital interaction.

We also thank our friends who endured our endless preoccupation with this book, and we hope they will feel that their patience was justified.

Our acknowledgements would not be complete without a heartfelt thanks to our husbands and daughters for their patient listening and encouragement, meals cooked, and our absences endured as they taught us that love is, indeed, a daily task.

Eugenie G. Wheeler & Joyce Dace-Lombard
April, 1989

CONTENTS

Publishers Notes

The purpose of this book is to give helpful guidelines to chronically ill people and their families. This publication is not designed to give medical information or psychological treatment. If medical care or counseling is needed, the services of a competent professional should be sought.

All the people profiled in this book are real people. Pseudonyms are used for the few who have requested anonymity.

FOREWORD
by

Robert E. Alberti, Ph.D.

"Courage," Mark Twain observed wisely, "is resistance to fear, mastery of fear--not absence of fear."

Courage of that sort is demanded every day from those who live with chronic illness -- not to mention considerable measures of patience, self-respect, and humor. Those qualities are not easily acquired or maintained. They require knowledge, skills, and continuing effort. *Living Creatively With Chronic Illness* provides access to the knowledge and skills--you'll have to supply your own effort.

As a psychologist and a publisher of self-help books (I did not, alas, publish this one!), I am acutely aware of the mythology and bad advice that is widely offered in the name of psychological self-help. This book suffers from neither shortcoming; it is not mythological, and it offers good advice. It's filled with sound ideas, well expressed. The book treats the subject of chronic illness comprehensively and with sensitivity, presenting an effective integration of facts, personal experiences of courageous people who suffer from chronic disease, and useful suggestions for self-help. The interviews with role models of chronic illness are done with empathy and depth, and the self-help procedures recommended are drawn from a wide variety of demonstrably valid approaches.

We should not be surprised that the authors of *Living Creatively With Chronic Illness* have done such a thorough job. Dace-Lombard and Wheeler are professionals who have extensive experience working with the chronically ill in a variety of settings. Their book is thoroughly researched yet practical and not too academic.

Living Creatively With Chronic Illness makes an important contribution to the lives of people suffering from chronic illness. I commend it to all who must resist and master the fears and challenges of a physical burden.

Robert E. Alberti, Ph.D.
Licensed Counseling Psychologist
Co-author, *Your Perfect Right*
President, Impact Publishers, Inc.
March 1989

INTRODUCTION

This book is about chronically ill people and how they cope with their unique problems as they move from being victims of circumstance, through becoming survivors, to transcending the pain, losses and frustration chronic conditions impose upon daily life. To transcend in this context means to go beyond, or rise above these impositions and focus on other aspects of living. It's about people who refuse to be devastated despite lost expectations, and who develop skills that bring them inner peace despite pain.

Chronic illness is different from either temporary or terminal illness. Coming to terms with the endlessness of chronic illness is different from coming to terms with finality.

The number of individuals who suffer from chronic illness is on the rise. This reflects not only the limitations of modern medicine but also to some degree the advances. People are able to live longer in spite of long standing ill health. Longer life spans and unhealthy environmental factors contribute to the incidence of chronic debilitating disease. The times we live in are reflected in the stories contained in these pages. Those who survived poliomyelitis in the 1950s are now found to develop many symptoms including recurrent weakness decades after their initial bout. On the other hand, young previously vital women are reporting elusive symptoms of what is being called a "yuppie disease," the chronic fatigue syndrome.

Everyone touched by chronic illness knows that life changes in all its aspects. Lifelong goals must be reassessed. Family relationships and roles may be drastically and irreversibly altered.

The opportunities or choices for work and play can become severely restricted. Personal family experiences with cancer, diabetes and rheumatoid arthritis have influenced the authors' understanding and sensitivity to the difficulties in adapting to life with chronic disease.

Part I of this book begins with the process of grieving as it applies to chronic illness. The information in this section will give you a road map through the territory of grieving losses, so that you can begin to move from feeling like a victim to becoming a survivor.

The second section addresses how you can go about restoring your sense of self. It includes profiles of people asking questions similar to yours and skill-building exercises to help you develop new strengths. As you deepen your understanding of the conditions that accompany chronic illness such as depression, pain, and fatigue, you can begin to counter them through building your self-esteem, developing the reflective skills necessary to understand yourself better, and building a basis of support through family, friends, and the larger world. This part validates that as you move from being a survivor to becoming a transcender, you set energy free to take action yourself, whether it be through celebrating small personal gains, or becoming an advocate or social activist for those who also suffer in some way.

The last part of the book is about living at your personal best. It's about turning points in your adjustments to chronic disease and about attitudes that help. It includes the healing power of spirituality, however you define it. The final chapter, **Soaring to Great Heights,** gives a mini-encyclopedia of the traits cultivated by people who are no longer merely surviving. To live at your personal best is to transcend victimization.

Guy Murchie in his book, *The Seven Mysteries of Life*, **defines transcendence in terms of time, space and self. Each aspect has to do with perspective and proportions. In terms of the self, there is a movement from the singular to the plural, from finitude to infinitude. Transcendence then is a widening of perspective. In**

relation to chronic illness it is being able to focus on aspects of life other than the illness.

This book is for you who have a chronic progressive illness. It primarily concerns chronically ill adults in their productive years who may or may not be bed-ridden, and do not necessarily have any visually discernible marks.

It is for you who are living daily with the pain and frustration of a disease that interferes with your daily living. In most cases these diseases are progressive, but not terminal--there is treatment, but no cure, no resolution or closure. Your disease may have presented symptoms which were separated from definitive diagnosis by months, or even years. It may have begun in childhood, or not until your teens, or in adulthood. There may have been remissions for weeks, months, or even years.

This book is for you who are touched by disease and impairment in "prime time," your productive years. It means that you are living within the context of building relationships with parents, children, colleagues, friends, or mates and finding meaning and purpose in your life. Prime time purpose and meaning may come from raising children, building a career, active volunteerism, being a student, or following an avocation. It does not necessarily mean being of "a certain age." Prime time vitality can be yours whether you're 16 or 70.

You may have people in your life who hurt and feel frustrated about how to help you live a happier, more productive life. They, too, are experiencing the losses, griefs, and adjustments that your chronic illness imposes on all of your lives. The chapter, **Understanding Your Family** offers helpful information about children, spouses, parents, siblings, and friends. By sharing this book with your family, you can use it as a springboard for improved communication and problem-solving. You can become a support system for each other.

While writing this book, the authors conducted surveys and led workshops for people with chronic illnesses such as multiple sclerosis, lung conditions, lupus, and arthritis. The authors learned from the many chronically ill people they interviewed--from the people who have commonly known conditions, and also from those whose conditions are less familiar, and who are breaking new ground in learning how to cope, and even grow. Interviews were conducted in offices, over the telephone, and in people's homes. The contributors to this book generously shared from the heart while the tape recorder silently recorded their concerns and insights. Some sent tapes across the country and lent papers they'd written.

The authors also learned about chronic illness from their many years of experience in clinics, hospital settings, teaching institutions and their own private practices. They are still learning and would like to hear from readers with suggestions for making possible future editions of this book even more helpful to people with chronic illness.

It takes information, motivation, skill, and support to accomplish the goals of transcendence. It has been said by the Danish philosopher, theologian Soren Kierkegaard that life can be understood backwards but must be lived forward. The following material can help you alleviate your pain, deepen your insights, and enhance your coping skills so that your life does indeed move forward to living creatively with chronic illness and transcending the pain.

PART I

LOST EXPECTATIONS

Part I is the shortest section of the book as it reflects the viewpoint that it is not helpful to dwell upon loss. However, to transcend your grief and pain, it is vital to address this ongoing aspect of living with a chronic illness.

It is helpful to learn that however individual your condition and problems may be, you are not alone. Others, from the rich and famous to the person living down the street from you, suffer.

In chapters one and two the ages of disease onset, and the stages you go through from denial of a serious condition, through feelings filled with protest and despair, to survivorship are discussed. The experience of family and friends is addressed briefly here; it is enlarged upon inPart II.

These beginning chapters provide a map of the territory. With this groundwork, the tools you use to cope make more sense, so that you can begin to transcend your diagnosis and condition.

IT'S IN THE LETTING GO

I felt a weight upon my chest
       -a leaden stone it seemed;
A child skipped by and caught my eye
       -tears spilled; I've been redeemed.
The lesson learned that quick spring day
       -just let the crack appear;
Left in the structure of a life
       remains all truly dear.
It's in the letting go of pain
       that wind borne seeds are strewn
And stronger roots are then sent down
       where once there was a ruin.
No need to be alone, my friend
       -your neighbor suffers, too.
The child skips by to catch our eye;
       -spring flowers plucked...so new.

                Joyce Dace-Lombard

1

YOU ARE NOT ALONE

High achieving role models can be intimidating as well as inspiring. The following heroes and heroines are worth knowing about, but don't let their greatness overwhelm you or make you feel anxious. You are not alone whatever the stage of your illness, or the level of your achievement.

Ludwig van Beethoven was condemned to total deafness. He defied the onset of despair with the "Eroica" symphony. It was believed that his deafness arose from chronic dysentery. The dysentery was relieved by treatment, but the deafness remained. His music, already sublime, moved into a new dimension as he possessed new and even greater powers as a composer.

Emily Dickinson, one of the most important woman poets of the United States, was in poor health and lived in seclusion. She wrote:

> We never know how high we are
> Till we are called to rise
> And then, if we are true to plan
> Our statures reach the skies.

Henri Matisse took up painting as a distraction while convalescing from an illness. Drawn to this new activity, he decided to dedicate himself to it completely.

Robert Louis Stevenson showed signs of pulmonary trouble even as a baby. When he was 23 his lung trouble declared itself in virulent form. At 28 he went to San Francisco poor and ill, lost his way en route to Monterey, and lay out in the open for three days and nights. This exposure did harm to his delicate constitution and he was an invalid for the rest of his life. But he still gave us *Treasure Island, Kidnapped*, and *Dr. Jekyll and Mr. Hyde*, living and working in the shadow of death.

Franklin Delano Roosevelt, thirty-second President of the United States and one of the greatest, the only one elected to four terms of office, was a polio survivor.

But it is not necessary to go back in history to find heroes and heroines of transcendence. Contemporary role models abound.

Otto Klemperer is a world renowned German conductor, now of the New Philharmonia Orchestra in London. Headaches tormented him after a fall from the podium in Leipzig. A medical checkup in Boston in 1939 revealed a brain tumor. Surgery was only partially successful for it left him with his right side paralyzed. Again in 1951 his career nearly ended because of injuries he suffered in a fall from a landing ramp at the Montreal Airport. A member of the Philharmonia in describing his conducting said, "Well, you see, it's as though Beethoven himself were standing there."

Actress Madlyn Rhue, who has multiple sclerosis, played the role of "Annie," a wheelchair-bound ballistic expert on the CBS television show, "Houston Knights."

Mary Tyler Moore, popular actress of television, stage, and screen, copes with diabetes.

Ann Ruth, a quadriplegic, is an artist and president of the Ann Ruth Greeting Card Company. She paints by holding the brush in her teeth.

Sefra Kobrin Pitzele, who has systemic lupus erythematosus, is the author of *We are Not Alone: Learning to Live with a Chronic Illness.*

Wendy Whiting, whose spastic cerebral palsy restricts her to a wheelchair, composes ballet. Though she is unable to perform the movements herself, she has dancers who, she says, "are helping to make my dreams come true, and put my emotions into motion."

You are not alone, moreover, even if you have not achieved greatness. Over 30 per cent of the adult population, or more than 55 million people, suffer from some form of one of the major chronic illnesses such as severe asthma, Parkinson's, impairing dystrophies, and cancer. Over 250,000 people in the United States suffer from multiple sclerosis, 2,000,000 from stroke with impairment, 4,600,000 from heart disease with impairment, and 11,000,000 from diabetes. You are not alone if you have a lung disease as there are 3,170,000 of you. According to some estimates there are 36,000,000 people with arthritis, and in that group over 7,000,000 have rheumatoid arthritis, 16,000,000 have osteo-arthritis, 2,000,000 have gout and 2,500,000 have ankylosing spondylitis. It can be confusing not only because estimates vary, but also because most of these major disease categories encompass several separate, discernable illnesses. For example, arthritis has some 100 identifiable forms.

These major, chronic, usually progressive diseases "attack" the different body systems: the immune, autoimmune, circulatory, and nervous system. They may "attack" the connective tissue such as skin, joints and muscle, or the vital organs, such as the kidneys, heart, lungs, pancreas and liver.

Besides the major chronic illnesses, lesser known ones exist such as Friedrich's ataxia (a neurological impairment), and newly defined chronic illnesses such as chronic fatigue syndrome, which is currently (1989) undergoing further medical definition. But this book is not about disease, it is about the people who have the diseases; the one out of every seven persons who lives with arthritis, and the one out of every twenty who lives with diabetes. The great majority of these people have not achieved fame, but many have transcended the pain of their illness successfully. In the chapter on taking social action you will meet Abby Spellman who transcends the disabilities of Freidreich's ataxia. In the chapter on pain and fatigue you will meet Sheila and Gisela, both diagnosed with chronic fatigue syndrome.

The disorganization that follows the crisis of chronic illness can be the beginning of a self-assessment that leads to more conscious development of deliberately selected traits. This is true of the people profiled in these pages.

But shock, anger, and fear are often the first feelings you experience upon diagnosis whenever it occurs, and so Part I is titled **Lost Expectations.**

Chronic Illness in Childhood

Your disease may have its roots in your childhood. Children with chronic illnesses and pain comprise ten to fifteen percent of the population of the United States. You might have grown up knowing that you were different from your friends: different in energy and stamina, different in how your body was growing and developing, different in your experience with disability and pain. This may have happened to you when you were very young, as a schoolchild, or during your teen years. It may have happened suddenly, with an illness, or over a long period of time with confusion and misdiagnosis, or as a slowly developing pattern of symptoms that began to grow into a diagnosis over months or years.

If you were chronically ill as a child, your questions might have included ones similar to those expressed in the following poem:

WHY MAMA?

Why can't I be like the other kids?
             run and play,
             laugh and swim
I only pout, and feel mad.
MAD 'cause I can't move as fast
             play as hard
             be as F R E E.
WHY?
Why can't I be like the other kids?
             whole of body,
             free of spirit,
 I only cry and feel sad.
SAD cause I can't join the fun
             keep a plan
             hone a skill.
WHY?
Why can't I be like the other kids?
             young when I'm young
             and old when I'm old.
 I can only hide and feel fear.

FEAR-'cause I'm confused and hurt.
             - I want to run.
             But run to where?

There's only your arms to hold me,
             your love to free me
             your hope to guide me.
Only in this safe port can I ask:

WHY MAMA?

                    Joyce Dace-Lombard

Kathleen Johnston-Cronk

Kathleen is an example of someone who contracted her illness in childhood. The love and support of her mother helped her feel safe and whole. She copes with multiple physical problems resulting from polio when she was four years old. As an adult, Kathleen transcended the physical limitations of post-polio syndrome by flying and riding horseback. She says, "Maybe I can't be a track star, but I learned to fly." And fly she did, whether it was in a small Piper cub adapted by her husband to accommodate a left foot that she can't depend upon, or on the back of a horse streaking over the countryside. She finds her wholeness in broader terms than her limbs. Restored, she is then able to focus her energies on her relationships, her work, and on being part of her community. She copes with the problems of illness--conflicts of dependence/independence--in her own way. She exudes spirit and courage, probably partly because she started to transcend some of the trauma of chronic illness even in childhood.

Chronic Illness in Adulthood

Your disease may have interrupted your adult years when you least expected such a discontinuity. Suddenly there is an end to a predictable sense about your life. You are not alone. Others in positions similar to yours have thoughts like this:

Once upon a time I knew what I could do tomorrow:
> *how fast I could run,*
> *how productively I could work,*
> *how quickly dinner could be prepared.*

Once upon a time I knew
> *how tightly I could hold you,*
> *how freely I could play,*
> *how I could spend Saturday evening -*
> *three weeks from now.*

Once upon a time I knew or thought I knew -
> *what work I could do,*
> *children I could bear,*
> *special person I would meet,*
> *what I would do in my middle years*
> *how I would look when I was seventy-five.*

And now, A F T E R:
> *after confusion*
> *after diagnosis*
> *after denial*
> *after tests run for whole days and weeks*

I only know how I feel right now
> *what I think right now*
> *what I can do, right now.*

Once upon a time has fallen down; been shattered
and "all the king's horses and all the king's men"
can't put the old me together again.

Joyce Dace-Lombard

With every new stage in your disease process, with every flare-up of symptoms, with every change, there is a temporary loss in your sense of self. If the "old me" can't be put back together again, you may ask yourself, "What is my task? To whom do I turn?"

Amye Leong

Amye Leong, who copes daily with the pain and frustration of rheumatoid arthritis, had the onset of her condition in adulthood. She has put herself "together again" after some false starts. Early in her years of living with the disease, when she was often in denial about the effects, she pushed herself too far and lost 20% of her body weight. She was in the hospital for 90 days, and into a three year flare up of symptoms. Since then she has learned the gentle art of living realistically with the arthritis while proceeding with an active and vital life. Her coping strategy begins with acknowledging that she must understand both the disease and herself. She knows that her positive attitude is a strength and that she uses denial at her own peril. She establishes limits and plans for successes that fall within her limitations. Amye has a successful marriage and works for a large company out of an office in her home. Restoring her sense of self is a daily task--she has strategies for coping with attitude and with physical frustrations. Amye has enough of herself left over to develop and facilitate a support group for young people living with arthritis. She makes a vital contribution to her chapter of the Arthritis Foundation. Amye has arthritis; arthritis does not have Amye.

Your path toward transcendence, like the illness with which you live, is an ongoing process with ongoing losses in expectations. You may transcend the pain, frustrations, and even boredom one day, just to feel defeated the next. This does not negate the fact that you have chosen to begin the process, or to "work the program." Just deciding to pursue this path, or even recognizing that you are taking the first steps toward it, is a transcendence in itself.

It is not possible to be transcending the losses and pain in all areas of your life all of the time. It is natural to feel a victim of your circumstances when you first receive distressing news. It is possible to be barely functioning as a survivor in some areas of your life, and yet be developing other aspects of yourself that transcend, or go beyond the catastrophe of disease. Stability finally comes from grieving losses, trusting in yourself, building coping skills, and gaining support. Growth comes from opening heart and soul to the experience of faith and restorative experience. This combination brings inner peace.

You Are Not Alone

2

LOSSES, GRIEF, AND ADJUSTMENTS

You may be familiar with the ancient legend of the Phoenix. This magical 500-year-old bird--so the story goes--took flight from Greece to Egypt. It entered the temple of Re, god of the sun, in the ancient city of Heliopolis, to fly into the flame of the fire lit by a holy priest. That would appear to be the end of the tale, but no; on the second day, a new form of life appeared in the ash; on the third day a magnificent bird rose from this place of desecration, taking flight toward the heavens.

What transforms this from a mere story into a legend is its universal appeal to people across time and cultures. It is a legend of resurrection. Out of the death of one form comes, unexpectedly, another.

Judith Viorst, in her best seller, *Necessary Losses*, addresses the *Loves, Illusions, Dependencies and Impossible Expectations That All of Us Have to Give Up in Order to Grow*.[1] People living with chronic and progressive illnesses often find their bodies aging prematurely, their health and lives in jeopardy. This requires an earlier than usual adaptation to certain kinds of change. In a chapter aptly titled "Shifting Images," Viorst writes, "we mourn the loss of our selves--of earlier definitions that our images of self depend upon. For the changes in our body redefine us. The events of our personal history redefine us. The ways that others perceive us redefine us. And at several points in our life we will have to relinquish a former self-image and move on."

What is the grief process in the lives of chronically ill people? Sheila finds that chronic fatigue syndrome leaves her too tired to call her near and dear friend. She no longer sees herself as having the boundless energy she expected to have indefinitely. Gone is the feeling that she is as resilient on the inside as she appears to be on the outside. When her symptoms flare up, self-care takes top priority. She's had to change her expectations--and her image--of herself.

Roger can no longer get down on the floor to wrestle with his eight year old son. The pain and immobilization of rheumatoid arthritis have made it necessary for him to change his companionship with the boy. They are now playing computer games, though sitting for long is also a difficulty. He has had to change his expectations about a father/son relationship.

Chronic illness for these people and for the others profiled in this book means a continued loss of expectation, and requires flexibility to adapt and change plans, sometimes daily. Unlike people living with a temporary or terminal illness, it won't be over. Daily life is often frustrating, and sometimes enraging. You suffer losses, you grieve, you cope, you grow.

People have always grieved their losses. Some of the most poetic literature across time and cultures speaks of sorrow. The Old Testament, literature from Judaism, Christianity, and the Eastern religions eloquently express bereavement, that state of being dispossessed of what is near and dear to one's happiness and wholeness. It is in the twentieth century, beginning with Freud, that strong human bonds, loss, and grief are understood so that informed support can be given to grieving people as they adjust. It is now known that grief has definable mental, emotional and physical aspects, and that a process of adaptation and recovery must take place over time. This process can be experienced, delayed, exaggerated, or seemingly absent. Psychiatrists such as Erik Lindemann, Colin Murry Parkes, John Bowlby, and Elizabeth Kubler-Ross provide the basis of what is now known. From their work you can see that grieving people move through stages during adjustment to loss. The following chart indicates these stages using two models:

ADJUSTMENT TO LOSS:	ACUTE GRIEF STAGE
KUBLER-ROSS	BOWLBY/PARKS
Stages to be experienced:	**Process; what's going on**
Denial	Denial/Shock/Numbness
Anger	Protesting the Loss
Bargaining	Yearning and Searching
Depression	Despair/Disorganization
Acceptance	Reorganization/Restoration

Resolution of acute grief

It is useful to understand these stages even though they may apply differently to chronic illness. There is no death of the body, but constant readjustment and therefore mourning for progressive losses.

The progress of your chronic illness is not orderly, structured, or conducted by following a set of instructions. There is uncertainty, unpredictability, and ambiguity. Again and again, you can go into remission, reach a plateau where reasonable stability can be anticipated, or go into a flare-up of symptoms. Coping can get tedious. Having to live like this is definitely not fair!

Stability in the face of chronic illness cannot come from following a neat guide on "Grief Resolution" in which you can anticipate a beginning, a middle and a resolution of grief. Stability must come from a trust in yourself, from grieving lost expectations, from building coping skills, from surrounding your self with support, and from reaching hitherto unknown inner resources. This combination can bring you inner peace, described by one woman who sustained a stroke as "a place of thanksgiving." Like the legendary phoenix, you must allow the parts of yourself that are no longer useful to die away so that a more encompassing self can be resurrected.

Before reaching inner peace, losses must be grieved, adjustments made, and a new self embraced. If you once ran marathons, that vital, athletic self must be grieved. If you once drove a car and must now be driven, that form of independence must be grieved. You will move yourself from victim to survivor as you grieve and begin to cope. Then you will move yourself from surviving to going beyond your illness, or transcending, as you begin to restore yourself within a larger definition of who you are.

A chronically ill person will experience two distinct processes of grieving in the journey through life. First, the feelings during the crisis of diagnosis or an escalation of symptoms, and secondly, the mourning of ongoing losses.

THE CRISIS PHASE

When a sudden onset of symptoms occurs, you and your family must cope with that crisis. Traditional or trusted ways of responding may not be enough. The task is to get through the immediate crisis. First of all, you will find yourself and those close to you stunned by shock and disbelief, followed by the desire to **do** something. After that a plethora of conflicting feelings will surface.

Stage 1: Shock, Disbelief, Denial

The phrase, "Life is what happens while you're making other plans" may apply. You might be building a career or making plans to have a child, go to school, buy a house, or take a trip. Then one day while running soapy hands over your body in the shower you linger over a lump that is still there after two months. Or you worry that the tingling sensation in your fingers just might be more than stress. Perhaps your spouse notices that you are bumping into things, and together you acknowledge something new and potentially frightening between you. Disbelief makes just a little room for acknowledgement but maybe not enough to get you to your doctor...yet.

Then one day you begin to face what's happening in your life and to the plans you've made. The trip can wait, but can the tests? You're beginning to end denial and enter an emotional crisis. You now want to **do** something. Perhaps in your case you didn't have the luxury of a slow realization that something was wrong. A sudden heart attack or stroke creates a clear clinical picture and quickly mobilizes family, friends, and treatment team into action. Although denial of the medical crisis is short-lived, denial of emotional, mental, or social losses may stretch on.

At other times, it can be months or even years between the disturbing appearance of symptoms and a definitive diagnosis. Often the afflicted person is the first in the family to know, down deep, that the problem is authentic. It's hard enough to know something's wrong yourself, and even more difficult when your family is afraid to face facts.

The length of time in this stage varies, depending upon the nature of the illness and the personalities of the people involved.

Stage 2: Mobilization to Action

Doing something usually helps people feel useful and is a way to cope with fear and anxiety. Often the threatened individual and the family respond quite differently at this time. The task of the person labeled "patient" is to survive, to control any growing panic, and to maintain a sense of self. Family members quickly separate themselves into "Doers" and "Retreaters."

Doers use their anxiety to mobilize themselves into action. They need to be in control, to take charge, so they gather information, do practical things, and act to protect the ill person. Although it is not apparent, these people will need support and help, too.

Retreaters are so overwhelmed by anxiety that they become either immobilized or leave. They need to regroup before they can take control. These people need support so that they can then become available to give support.

You may recognize some of your family members, or even yourself, in these descriptions. It helps if there is someone such as a friend, counselor, or religious advisor who can be an advocate for the family while you are all in crisis.

Stage 3: Dealing with Feelings and Thoughts

During the time that the crisis is being managed, a wealth of feelings and thoughts occur. Overriding feelings are usually fright and apprehension. You or a family member may feel "frozen." The fight/flight anxiety response is at work. There is a drive to do and act, yet at the same time you want to run away from the crisis. Some people run, some stay and cope, some are immobilized. Hearts pound, palms sweat, blood pressure rises, muscles contract, adrenalin flows, just as in earlier times when there was a tiger to fight. A real, live beast seems so much easier to fight! You may feel helpless, have many self doubts, and say all kinds of things that begin with "shoulds" and "oughts." You and your family may think and/or say things like: "I should have noticed those symptoms sooner," or "Why didn't I make you stop smoking, knowing there were heart attacks and strokes in your family?" or "If only we hadn't been under so much stress..." You alternate between blame and fear as you try to get a handle on yourself at this time of crisis.

Stage 4: Resolution of Crisis

You cannot return to your pre-crisis situation, since a chronic medical condition will now have to be managed. The hoped for outcome is an understanding of the nature of your disease, and a better understanding of yourself. This book will give you a guide to help you to identify issues, develop coping skills, and get on with your life. During a crisis it is understandable that you feel like a victim, and that your family feels victimized. As you move into mourning ongoing losses, you will have the time and energy to develop coping skills and find support. You will find the resources within yourself to survive.

ONGOING LOSSES:

This will be an overview of your losses as you adjust to long-term change. Your family's feelings and adjustments are discussed in Chapter 5, **Understanding Your Family**.

When your are living with a chronic illness you live with loss on a daily basis. A person with diabetes loses the luxury of spontaneity where food and activity are concerned. One's social life may become regimented by the need to balance daily metabolic requirements. People with diseases of the cardiovascular, musculoskeletal or nervous systems may have a loss of ability to keep up with the demands of sudden exertion and mobility needed for work or play. If asthma is a life threatening condition for you, unsolicited advertisements containing fragrant samples arriving in the mail constitute a major threat to your health. No matter what your condition, restrictions exist. What is a mere annoyance for many--perhaps for your family--is critical for you. Your anger is a part of your ongoing grief. When you lose your freedom, choice, and spontaneity you experience a huge loss.

Denial

At first, as you begin to get on with your life, you will try to deny the severity of the restrictions. You will test the reality. You may wake up in the morning temporarily forgetful of your limitations. Although you now have a diagnosis and perhaps a prognosis with which to grapple, you face this with relief mixed with dread. Relief, because you can now develop a game plan; dread, because you were hoping against all odds that it wasn't true. You may tempt fate, push the odds, and seem like your old self to your family. Your head may tell you one thing while your gut is saying another.

Anger and Other Feelings

But soon--sooner than you'd like--the feelings begin to flow. You protest your outrage. Like a wounded animal you cry out; like a frightened child you lash back. You may feel betrayed by God. And oh, the jealousy directed toward those more able-bodied. You may feel trapped in a failing body, humiliated by the extent of your inadequacies, surprised by your vulnerability, and angered and saddened by the loss of a youthfully responsive body. Perhaps you are heartsick over the threat to your spontaneity, and at being treated unfairly by a demanding and far-from-benevolent culture. A part of you is searching for the "old me"; a part of you is struggling with cutting your losses and getting on with it, though it would help if you knew what "it" is going to be.

Along with all of these feelings is the constant chatter in your head, much of it the voice of guilt: "Why didn't I take better care of myself? Will anyone ever love me again? Why didn't I appreciate my body more when I was well?"

Bargaining

Along about this time, you find yourself striking bargains with God, even if you were one of those professed "God is Dead" proponents of a youthful rebellion. "Just let me get through school...or see the children launched...or have five good years to do everything I want to do in my lifetime," you plead. The anger, the bargaining, the myriad feelings and thoughts are attempts to get your old self back again. They are the protest against loss, the yearning and searching for your familiar self.

Depression, Sadness, Isolation

Now in place of the searching is depression. It is natural that you are depressed when you can no longer deny what is happening, when you are tired of the struggle against limitations. While earlier you wanted to be heard by your compatriots, now you seek solitude. Alone to think, you manage to regroup. You begin to restore your sense of self which must be incorporated into the "new me." In this quietude, you begin to assess your losses and your life. This encompasses every area, the physical, emotional, mental, financial, social, and spiritual. This is a large task and will be accomplished in pieces, over time. Everyone has a picture within themselves of how they imagine themselves to be. By the time you are an adult, you have formed a unique perception of your physical being. You know what you think and feel about things and people. You have an idea of what kind of work you will do and how much money you'll make. There is a workable way in which you relate to people. These thoughts, feelings and perceptions form your values. Your ideals about yourself and your life will be challenged as you continue to cope with your illness. It takes time to reassess your life, to sort out what is still useful and to mourn the loss of what is not. This is a quiet, reflective time.

What to Think About During this Reflective Time:

Several aspects about you and your family influence the ease with which you grieve, let go, and begin to cope. Ask yourself the following questions and see if your answers give you any insight into where you will need to work the hardest:

- How well do I trust? (If you had trouble trusting your parents, or other important people, you may have trouble trusting yourself and the significant people in your life now).

- How independent or dependent am I? (A healthy mix will help you toward interdependence).

- How flexible am I? How willing am I to let go of out-worn attitudes or roles?

- Can I identify and communicate my feelings?

- Can I identify my previous coping skills and transfer them to this new situation?

- To what degree have I found satisfaction in my life prior to the onset of illness? (Grieving for what never was, nor ever will be, is difficult at best, and hardest for those least satisfied with their lives).

Other Serious Concerns

When you have a demanding job to do, such as adjusting to a chronic illness, you may find one or more "Red Flags" popping up. These are areas of concern that may need the attention of a professional person, such as a counselor. Go over the following list of danger signals. If you answer "yes" to any one, you will need to follow up with further investigation.

- Do you see yourself as stuck in any one feeling or thought, such as anger or blame?
- Do you think you are denying the reality of your incapacities longer than you, or others, consider reasonable?
- Are you resisting following medical advice to the detriment of your health?
- Are you creating other physical problems?
- Do you have low levels of contact with people, i.e., do you live alone, not work, or not do much socializing?
- Are there other major changes occurring in your life such as divorce, children leaving home, or ill parents ?
- Do you have a history of anxiety or depression that lasted longer than several months?
- Have you ever been treated medically for anxiety or depression?
- Have you ever thought about suicide to the extent that you developed a plan?
- Do you feel that there isn't even one person you can really talk to?
- Do you lack meaningful work, people, and activities in you life?
- Are your family and friends expressing undue concern about you?

If you checked off even one of these "Red Flags," it is important that you talk about these issues in your life with a concerned individual, perhaps a professional. By approaching these areas as problems to be solved, you will help move yourself from the role of victim to that of a survivor.

Feeling Better: Reaching a Level of Acceptance

There comes a time when you feel better about yourself and your life. Although you will cycle through the feelings and thoughts of loss and grief again, you will find that you don't fall as hard nor stay down as long. You will have developed coping skills and found support for yourself and your family.

Your picture of grief may look like this:

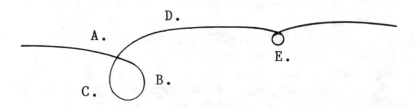

A. Original crisis, or escalation of symptoms, initially disbelief, shock and denial.

B. Going into action: myriad feelings and thoughts.

C. Depression, sadness, a time of inner regrouping.

D. Restoring your sense of self, feeling better. Note: you will leave the cycle at a higher level of coping than you entered.

E. Later cycle of grief.

Although you begin as a victim of disease, you become a survivor by learning to cope. As you develop a new sense of yourself, your life transcends the disease with which you live. Eleanor Roosevelt said, "Go down and answer up if you can...it's not easy." The life adjustments of Burt and Marsha Danet illustrate what this means.

Marsha and Burt Danet

Marsha and Burt Danet have contended with progressively more serious disability over the last 20 years. It began with an automobile accident when she was 23 and he 27. As a result of the injuries, a neurologist said to her that she must consider herself a semi-invalid. Marsha says, "The healthy part of me said to him, 'Well, if I'm a semi-invalid, then by definition I'm semi-healthy. I want to deal with the semi-healthy and I'm going to let you deal with the semi-invalid.' He thought I was denying. I knew there were many more qualities to me than my injured spine."

Marsha and Burt were in several automobile accidents over the next twenty years. Various forms of arthritis have settled into the areas of injury for Marsha. Together they both suffer from exquisitely painful neurological and orthopedic symptoms. Both have been diagnosed as having myofascial pain syndrome, also commonly called fibrositis syndrome. Myofascial pain syndrome is characterized by migratory pain and stiffness of the musculoskeletal system associated with skin and muscle tenderness. Poor quality, restless sleep is part of the symptomatology seen in this condition.

The Danets, like all who are confronted with chronic illness, have gone through stages of grief, mourning and depression. In Burt's words, "There is definitely a reaction that you have to go through to cope with and deal with what you're facing. We have this notion that as you go through life you are not supposed to have these things happen to you. And then they do happen, and now you're faced with it. You think you're supposed to live a life free of pain. Who ever said that? No one ever said that. Maybe part of what is natural in living is that some of us develop pain--that that's part of the way it is. Maybe we have to take that into account."

The dreams they have had to give up span all areas of their lives. He is a psychologist. She had planned to return to school. They planned to work in the field of psychology together. Instead they are co-editors and publishers of a newsletter, **The Health**

Examiner: Gold Coast Edition. They are providing leadership for a project called "Partnerships for a Better Community." On the masthead of their publication is the slogan, "Striving For The Best Within Us." From the outside that doesn't look so hard, for there is no outward physical evidence of major impairment. Only Burt sees the splints Marsha puts on her arms to give them a rest. A postman who is fond of them, and who often slaps her on the shoulder, doesn't see the disability or the sharp pain his affectionate gesture causes her.

But Marsha is aware of the changes. She describes herself as once young and vibrant. Now she tells of the time she viewed herself in the full-length mirror of their bedroom, saw her bent over appearance, found it comical, and roared with laughter. "Later I cried," she said, "because it was also sad, but it was funny, too." Her playfulness and spontaneity are intact.

Changes in body image are sometimes addressed at unplanned moments. Several months after the previous incident, Marsha walked past a plate glass mirror in a shopping center and saw what appeared to be a disabled person behind her. Marsha arrived at the door and turned to allow the person to pass in front of her, only to discover that the image she'd seen was her own. Losses in self image are experienced as they come up, which can be anywhere, any time. These are just as real as losses of mobility.

Both Marsha and Burt have lost their sense of a safe, secure world, their freedom from pain, their earlier sense of themselves and their earlier expectations. It would be easy for such people to lose their sense of humor and spontaneity, but quite the opposite is true of the Danets. Humor and spontaneity have become coping mechanisms. Their dreams of working together are being fulfilled; only the vehicle is different. It has been out of their pain and suffering that their involvement in creating a better community has occurred. Perhaps some of their success is due to Marsha's attitude. She refuses to call what happened to her and her husband a problem; she refers to it as a challenge.

NOTES

PART II

RESTORING YOUR SENSE OF SELF

This section addresses some of the unique problems that you as a person with a chronic illness face and suggests how you might handle them. Countering depression, coping with pain and fatigue, understanding your family, and maintaining your self-esteem are all key factors in learning to live with chronic illness. Other suggested approaches for restoring your sense of self are developing reflective skills, reaching out for support, taking social action, and learning to celebrate even small gains.

Each new skill you gain makes you less of a victim and more of a survivor. These steps aren't sequential in the sense that, once you have mastered a skill, you never have to go back and reprocess or learn new ways to handle problems. However, the suggested strategies you choose, whether they involve assertive communication skills or imaging, art or social action, will help you with your daily coping. As you practice them, you will find yourself growing inwardly. New facets of your personality will develop, and you will progress toward transcendence.

THE AUTHOR OF MY LIFE

I am the author of my life,
The success and failures,
The joys and strife.
I audition characters every day
And decide which will go
And which will stay.
Yes, I am the author of the play.

The setting is also mine to choose.
The setting of mountain, city or sea,
That decision rests upon me.
Comedy, epic or tragedy.

I decide what the leading person should be,
The leading person, of course, is me.
Hours and hours I rehearse
To make that character
A blessing or a curse.
So give this idea some thought today,
And you be the author of your play.

Nicholas Lentine1[1]

3

COUNTERING DEPRESSION

Depression is virtually inevitable in the process of coming to terms with a chronic illness. Different perceptions of depression lead to different responses to it. To some people, depression is such a natural and healing response to loss that they choose at first to stay with it rather than counter it. Included in this chapter are profiles of two people who counter their depressions successfully. Joyce Kisheneff is a counselor, and Belinda is an artist who uses artistic expression, such as painting, sculpture and poetry, as outlets, or channels, for her pain.

However, if after employing some of the skills presented in this chapter, you still find that your symptoms persist, it is important that you discuss it with your doctor. If your depression is lasting for months, and is seriously interfering with your daily life, it is wise to see a trusted therapist or doctor and have it evaluated for treatment and possible medical intervention. Only you can determine, based on your experience and philosophy about depression, which approach you wish to explore. You should be aware that some forms of depression are organic in origin, and respond to medical intervention. On the other hand, depression can also be a side effect of some medications you might be taking. With some diseases depression is part of the syndrome. These are all reasons why persistent symptoms of depression should be discussed and evaluated by your doctor. Another helpful way to view depression is to see it as a clue that not enough of your needs are being met. This puts you in a problem-solving stance and helps you take responsibility to find need-meeting resources and to make choices. When you realize that you have options and can make choices, you regain lost personal power and, consequently, feel better about yourself.

Sometimes it seems that no choices are left when you face the restrictions imposed upon you by your illness, especially since chronic illness, at least initially, generates feelings of discouragement and downheartedness. That's when it's important to realize that alternatives do exist to the way you view and respond to your problems. Knowing how different schools of thought define depression and the varying approaches they use to work with it can provide you with lots of strategies to employ when your options seem limited.

One school of thought, first espoused by Freud, describes depression as anger turned inward upon the self. This passive response keeps it inside and can create emotional and physical problems. On the other hand, anger acted on aggressively and irresponsibly can get you into all kinds of trouble. The solution is to direct your anger outwardly in a non-destructive manner. Acquiring the communication skills to express your anger assertively also improves your self-esteem and relationships. (This approach to anger-management is discussed in more detail in Chapter 7, **Maintaining Self-Esteem.**) Skillful management of anger is critical when you are suffering with a chronic condition because it is so easy to project the anger you feel at being disabled onto those who are treating your illness or onto those you love.

A behavior modification approach to depression views it as a drop in positive reinforcers. Perhaps you miss the workout of a tennis game, the camaraderie of the work place, or the strokes you received from a more active social life. It takes self-love, motivation, energy, imagination, and assertive skill to find compensation for these losses. It also takes courage to ask for help to meet these unmet needs in new ways. These are difficult skills to learn, so have patience with yourself!

Another perception of depression is "learned helplessness." This means that no matter how hard you try, you still do not have any impact on your environment. Some experts think that the origins of childhood depression occur when parents don't pay any attention to their child no matter what he or she does. Thus the child has no impact on the world and "learns" a feeling of pervasive helplessness. The person simply gives up on making choices. Learned helplessness is also characteristic of hostages, prisoners, and others who cannot influence what is happening to them. It is a victim's position.

Is it any wonder that when your autonomy is threatened by chronic illness, you, too, are at risk of feeling all the symptoms of learned helplessness? As you move forward from the original crisis of diagnosis, you can continue to be controlled by your illness, or you can recognize your choices in order to control those elements of your life that are controllable. For example, you can use your imagination and assertive skills to remain in charge of your life, as do the two women who are profiled at the end of this chapter. Both of them have often been angry and depressed, but they have chosen to use many resources, including therapy, to regain a sense of self. They have employed a wide range of skills, especially artistic expression, to achieve a sense of purpose.

Victor Frankl,[2] a well-known psychiatrist, while imprisoned in a concentration camp, became fascinated with the question of why some people became survivors and others did not. Although "fate" unquestionably played a part in the deaths of millions, he observed that survival had less to do with constitutional vigor than with a sense of purpose. Frankl concluded that a depressed will and depressed energy reflected a loss of meaning and a loss of purpose. It was the ability to keep a sense of purpose in the midst of a seemingly senseless world that created survivors out of potential victims. Frankl's philosophy and his very life are testaments to the fact that one can suffer, survive catastrophic losses, and affirm and celebrate life in the midst of disaster. The antidote to depression from this viewpoint, then, is to reassess your current goals and purpose and use what energy you have available to set appropriate new goals, to create new purpose.

In setting new goals, it helps to structure time so that you have three things to look forward to: something today, such as a phone call to a friend, or a special T.V. show, something within a few weeks or months, such as a holiday activity or a visitor, and something longer term. The important thing is not whether these exact goals are realized, but that they get you through some rough spots and generate hope. Structuring time in itself can alleviate the depressing feeling that things are going to stay bad indefinitely. Goal-lessness leads to boredom and irrelevance. Goal setting creates meaning and purpose. Start where you are; a long journey begins with a single step.

The famous Swiss psychoanalyst, Carl G. Jung, developed an analytical psychology based on his belief that the unconscious contains moral and religious principles. Depression develops from a disharmony between the ego, or the self we **think** we are, and the parts of ourselves we don't know we are, the collective unconscious. The goal is to be in touch with the unconscious, and self-understanding on this level <u>requires</u> depression--a slowing down--to work through it. Depression was thus perceived by Jung as a place and time of "waiting upon," or experiencing fully whatever you are feeling.

People who subscribe to this viewpoint stay with the depression with guidance, to learn from it. When you do this you will find this mood state acceptable, for this time of depression can be a period for inner growth and nurturance of the soul.

Another psychiatrist, Otto Rank, defined depression as blocked creativity. In fact, it is hard to imagine being creative and being depressed at the same time. That's when activities such as occupational therapy, a leisure-time class, wood carving, or solitary stitchery can contribute to your life. Capitalizing on a spontaneous creative impulse can also free you from a depressive grip, so give in to that impulse to take a walk, to plant a six-pack of flowers, to write something, or to play the piano. Anything that you perceive as creative, that will unblock your creative juices, is an antidote to depression.

For some people, this creativity is used to benefit others. They form new affiliations, or take social action. An example is Dianne Piastro who recognized that many young single adults who have a disability feel especially deprived because of having to curtail their social activities. She set up a dating service, "Special Connections," that focuses on matching singles who are physically disabled or have health challenges. The questionnaires ask not only the typical dating service questions, but also what members are willing to accommodate in a relationship (wheel chair, walker, crutches, cane, pacemaker, artificial limb, seeing eye dog, etc.) One woman had circled that she didn't want to meet a man in a wheel-chair because her first husband had been very dependent on her and she didn't want that again. Ms. Piastro told her about a man in a wheelchair who sounded quite independent. The woman gave it a chance, and now they've got a nice friendship going.[3]

Another definition of depression is that all depression is oppression. Of course this is simplistic, but while you are assessing the elements of your depression, you might consider if you are being, or are feeling, oppressed by the thoughtless attitudes of others toward people with physical impairments. If you've been subjected to insults through being stared at, being called a "cripple," or being put down in some way, it is important that you counter such an assault on your sense of self. Internalized put-downs lower self-image and erode self-esteem, and aggressive rejoinders don't usually get you very far (except into trouble). Assertive responses, again, both help to educate and to put you in charge of the situation.

At the least, depression should be taken as a clue that something is out of balance, that needs are not being met, that your usual coping strategies are not sufficient to meet the changes that occur between your former existence and the restructuring of your life into a newer, emotionally stronger one. As you formulate your own beliefs about your self, you may well come to view your depressed moods--and coping styles--as a composite of several of the above systems of belief, for they are not mutually exclusive.

Following are stories of two women, each of whom carved out her own individual way to counter depression.

Joyce Kisheneff[4] Ms. Versus M.S. (Multiple Sclerosis)

At the age of 42, Joyce was no ordinary graduate of a Master's program in psychology. She had multiple sclerosis and lacked the control and coordination necessary to walk, and couldn't see without shutting one eye. In 1988, she was a candidate for a doctoral degree and has been practicing successfully as a licensed therapist specializing in drug abuse and eating disorders.

How did Joyce learn to accept this incurable and progressive disease and become a productive human being? She believes that she learned the fighting tools from her mother, an insulin dependent diabetic who always told her, "Let's make lemonade out of a lemon." She has done just that with her life.

Joyce was stricken with multiple sclerosis at the age of 27. Multiple sclerosis is a chronic degenerative disease of the nervous system. Loss of function of crucial areas of the brain and spinal cord can occur. The course of multiple sclerosis can be extremely variable. Some individuals may have rapidly progressive loss of function while others may have years of slowly progressive or even apparently inactive disease. This variability can lead to considerable anxiety and depression since doctors often cannot predict the individual's future level of functioning. In Joyce's case, as in most others, she experienced attacks and remissions. Each attack left her with more disability on her left side and more visual problems. She also experienced frequent spells of weakness, numbness, pins-and-needles sensations, double vision and blurred speech.

When the first symptoms of M.S. appeared, her husband, Harry, was horrified. "I can't believe it, but whatever it is, we'll live with it together," Harry told her. Although he had never had any contact with a progressive illness, Harry accepted many new responsibilities, including helping with household chores.

Their son, Stephen, now 25 and finishing his last year of medical school, learned of Joyce's disease when he was only four years old. "Are you ever going to get better, Mom?" he asked. She tried to explain as best she could that her disease was not curable and was not going to go away.

Like many victims of incurable diseases, Joyce had difficulty adjusting to a new way of life. She had many lessons to learn. Luckily, she found supportive psychotherapy helpful in dealing with her anger toward her disease and the lack of diagnostic procedures and treatment remedies for the symptoms she was experiencing. Expressing her anger and staying in therapy led her to an entirely different and ultimately rewarding life. She realized she would have to find new areas of exploration and gratification.

"Therapy helped me research the resources that remained in spite of my illness," Joyce says. "I focused on how to get the most out of life, often in the face of obstacles which seemed to make my life feel impossible at times. I learned I was finding it very easy to complain to friends and loved ones about the horrible disease. I found that I almost enjoyed complaining. Therapy taught me to limit these complaints to the doctor's office.

"I learned it was okay to depend on friends and neighbors and I lost my inhibition about asking them to help me. A dear friend said, 'You can't just lie there and feel sorry for yourself. I'll take you to the market and to school.' I let her do it. I found that people enjoy making others happy, and if they can help you, they help themselves, too. I learned not to be ashamed of being first in movie lines or at Disneyland because, if given a chance, people understand my problems."

As a college student, Joyce had many problems to solve. Double vision forced her to listen to taped texts instead of reading. Neurological problems forced her to learn to pace herself through the day. Her doctors told her that bedrest during the attacks might minimize the progression of her disease, so she made herself lie down two to three hours in the afternoon. If out shopping, she would find a bench and sit down to rest for a while.

Depression is frequently associated with M.S. When it occurs, Joyce tries to leave the house, if only for a few hours, and is thus able to avoid arguments and aggravation. Often she goes out for lunch and comes back renewed. When she can't seem to get away, she has a massage or takes the vitamin medication prescribed by her doctor to calm her nerves. Joyce says,

> *I have had to learn to find happiness by being able to control my life as best I can. I became susceptible to infections and had to spend many days in bed. Any cold or virus can aggravate my illness. I have to be very careful. During these times I have someone help with the housework. I've learned fluent Spanish so I can communicate with my housekeeper.*

> *Exercise is very important for me. I need to use the weakened muscles in order to keep them from getting even worse.*

The greatest help in constructing and adjusting to her new life came from her husband and son. They encouraged her to find things to do that she could enjoy. Over a period of twenty years she has slowly moved ahead and has achieved great happiness in conducting her private counseling practice and in seeing her son become a doctor.

In describing her philosophy Joyce says,

> *Despite the tragedies a person may face, there is a bright side just waiting to be found. Multiple Sclerosis has not destroyed my intelligence or reasoning ability. I live one day at a time....Now, more than ever, I want to see and*

*feel things and find out what we are all about as people.
I relish my roles as therapist, teacher, lecturer, wife, and
mother. I am happy. I am.*

Belinda: Poetry out of Pain

Belinda has also developed effective measures for countering depression. She had a stroke in 1981 and also suffers from lupus erythematosus and arthritis. Art is Belinda's outlet and her therapy, the activity that gives her life meaning and restores her sense of self. She paints and does wood sculpture and collages, although sometimes her hands and back hurt her so much that she has to stop.

There have been times when even art and her considerable inner strength have failed her. Then she has turned to poetry, a medium in which she is also talented. She sometimes expresses her feelings of desperation in this manner. It is as if she pulls the poetry out of her pain, and it is a step toward her regaining hope, especially when it comes to "second victimizations." This term is used to describe hardships stemming from the illness, but going beyond it and compounding it such as side effects of medications, stigma, or lawsuits.

To be ill is difficult enough, but in addition there can be financial deprivations, perhaps long waits at clinics and seeing a different doctor-in-training at every visit. (Sometimes they give you different diagnoses, too.) Belinda is appreciative of the medical care that she receives, but seldom sees the same physician more than once, and it was quite a while before her self-diagnosis of stroke was confirmed. Instead her complaints were "pooh-poohed." She has also suffered the side effects of various medications and has to explain repeatedly that she is sensitive to many drugs.

Belinda's worst ordeal was her twenty-month struggle for S.S.I. eligibility, (Supplemental Security Income.) Then, after ten months' eligibility, she was declared well enough to return to work. She refers to the hearings as her "Nuremburg Trial." The following poem expresses her feelings and those of many who,

41

like Belinda, have to go through similar suspenseful and demeaning ordeals, on top of their disease impairments, to attain the wherewithal to survive.

THE HEARING

There's nothing like the truth
To clear your head
When life has been living illusions
Perceived with unspoken dread.

Feeling your mind dissolving
Pieces flying behind closed eyes
Lost dreams, ambitions, trust
Even hope, all go dashing by.

There's nothing like the truth
Unvarnished--naked and unkempt
To blast you to reality
To leave the dream undreamt.

Intrusions into privacy
Papers unfolded, discussed and filed
Present you are there
Body soiled--now mind defiled.

There's nothing like the truth--lastly
To unwind spirit from the mind
Spoken of as in the third person
Mutely limboed--now also blind.

With nothing left to cover
From the grudging, baneful eye
I stand here now--diminished--exposed
And idly left to die.[5]

Belinda is a stunning looking woman in her early fifties, an artist who wears clothing and jewelry that set off her beautiful coppery hair and her tall, willowy figure. When one talks with her about subjects other than her illnesses, it is difficult to believe that this woman has been through so many trials.

After her stroke she found it necessary to take on a partner in her antique business. Belinda did well, despite her physical difficulties, until the loss of the lease left her at loose ends. She decided to lease some shopping mall property, but when the city tore up the street in front of the building and made access almost impossible for months and months, she was forced into bankruptcy. Belinda still feels this was a reflection on her own integrity, even though she did everything in her power to make the business work.

However, Belinda was courageous then as she is now. She went "cold selling" - designing and painting murals in homes and businesses, selling at swap-meets, trying everything she could to keep afloat financially, but her weakness and loss of balance worsened. There was a two year downhill slide after the stroke which included the pain of the later diagnosis of lupus.

Systemic lupus erythematosus or lupus is an immune system disease. The immune system which normally helps fight off infection begins producing factors which inflame and can injure many organs of the body. The joints and skin are commonly involved but lupus may attack the kidneys, muscles, lungs, nervous system, heart and even blood cells. There are two common forms of lupus, discoid and systemic. Discoid lupus is a more limited form of the disease that involves primarily the skin. Belinda has the more serious, systemic form of the disease. She finally had to stop doing the murals after several falls from the home-made scaffolding she assembled. She couldn't afford, nor could she physically handle, professional steel scaffolding.

Countering Depression

Belinda took five courses at a community college recently. She continues to make collages and sculptures, does art criticism for a local paper, attends art shows when she is physically able, and writes poems. These are her creative ways of countering her depression.

STEPS YOU CAN TAKE TO COUNTER DEPRESSION:

- Identify some of the strategies that Joyce and Belinda use to counter depression. What assertive actions have they taken? What creative outlets have they devised?

- Note both your passive and aggressive responses toward yourself and toward other people. Note assertive "take charge" responses. Reward yourself for your successes with little things, like a good book or your favorite food. Assertive responses counter depression.

- Review your life, starting with your childhood, to uncover patterns of learned helplessness.

- Keep a tally which shows you the old reinforcers that you have lost, and the new ones that you are putting into place. Keep building new ones.

- Assess your life up to this point as to what has held meaning and purpose for you. Write down anything that has a new meaning, or the potential for meaning.

- Give yourself a goal for today, for later this week, and for a month from now. You can change your goals if you choose. The important thing is to have events to look forward to. Write them down.

- Do something creative **today**. It may be planned, or spontaneous, minute or large. Just **do** it.

NOTES

4

COPING WITH PAIN AND FATIGUE

People living with chronic conditions usually experience a cluster of symptoms--pain and fatigue often lead the list. Pain is perceived differently by different people, and it occurs in several forms.

It may be helpful to you in your pain management plan if you think about the many components of pain and suffering. The antidote to each is different. The hoped for outcome is comfort, or the release from suffering.

Organic pain is the physical pain that is part of your condition, a protective mechanism that tells you something is wrong and alerts you to seek medical intervention. Pain can be acute, with a beginning and an end, or it can be chronic which means that it has no set time limits. Chronic pain has a never-ending quality that requires special skills and perseverance to transcend. Organic, or physical pain is affected by all of the other kinds of pain--mental, emotional, social, and spiritual.

Mental pain reflects your attitude and other thoughts. Perceptions of mental pain vary greatly among people depending upon how they learned about pain and suffering when they were young. Jeanne Naspo, who developed juvenile rheumatoid arthritis when an infant, before she could understand pain, describes it this way:

> *My mother knew how to take the pain away. She acknowledged it, she nurtured me, she diverted my attention by telling me stories, she worked me through it. Her loving care countered any bitterness I might have developed.*

Now Jeanne at 37 has this attitude:

> *I respect pain, and I have learned discipline and courage. When the pain is gone, I am a free woman, and there isn't* **anything** *I can't do!*

Your mental attitude is a strong component in how your pain affects you. It is reflected in the degree to which you suffer Consider whether a change in your **perception** of pain can be a tool for change in your life. **Emotional pain** is inextricably related to physical pain. Emotional pain, particularly fear and rage, causes bodily changes which in turn can cause stress. Conversely, emotions such as hope and laughter create an environment for healing.

Social pain is significant, too; fatigue and loss of bodily functions can lead to loss of relationships, the loss of affiliation. This, in turn, can bring the suffering of alienation and loneliness.

Spiritual pain is the anguish you feel when life temporarily loses its meaning. It exaggerates your physical pain.

PAIN AND DEPRESSION

Pain does not exist in a vacuum. The various kinds of pain are part of a downward-spiralling cycle of experience which looks like the table on the following page:

PAIN -- DEPRESSION CYCLE

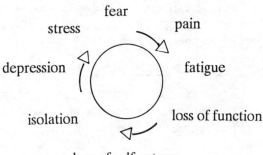

Although you can enter the cycle at any point, entrance often occurs when you fear pain. This can be the onset of the physical pain of inflamed joints, or the mental underlying fear that your condition will worsen. Pain creates strong emotions, too, which are also painful, and the cycle has to be worked through if you are to move on to a positive attitude. Intervening in this cycle by taking action helps you maintain your self-esteem and counter depression.

Fatigue

Fatigue is another unwanted companion of chronic illness-- the kind that is incomprehensible to those who do not live with it. Coping with the constant presence of fatigue is in itself fatiguing, for it means planning a day with the precision of a chef creating a special meal. It requires constant monitoring and choice making. To a person in a lupus or rheumatoid arthritis flare, or to someone living with chronic fatigue syndrome, it may mean preparing for and working a three-hour day and then lying on the couch at home for five hours. There is no energy left to wash your hair, visit with a friend, or prepare dinner. When fear and pain are added to this low energy level it is no wonder that your self-esteem goes down. If you have little self-esteem, if you remain in a morass of despair for any long period of time, social isolation is the inevitable outcome. When the natural need for healthy solitude turns sour, it, in turn, can lead to a deep and pervading depression. If this negative cycle becomes entrenched, it adds even more stress, which creates more fear and pain...and on...and on... Stress becomes distress.

INTERVENTIONS IN THE PAIN - DEPRESSION CYCLE

In seeking a way out of suffering, some people use pills, alcohol, or tranquilizers. Others become increasingly passive. None of these attempts provides lasting relief, and they all keep you a victim of your condition. A better way to start is to ask questions like the ones Leo Buscaglia poses in his book *Person-hood*,[1] "What is this hurt about? What is there for me to learn from it? What are my alternative responses besides suffering?"

Imagery

One alternative response is the use of imagery, which can be extremely effective in helping you live with chronic pain. Imaging gives a sense of mastery as you use fantasy to trigger relaxation. Through relaxation, endorphins, the body's natural tranquilizers, are released. Three people who have developed this skill imaginatively to cope with pain are Marsha, Ken, and Barbara.

Marsha, who suffers from chronic muscle pain, uses a form of imagery called disassociation. Once, while in a grocery checkout line, she was in unbearable pain and felt trapped. She chose a creative and unconventional response; she mentally sent her body outside the store, floating on a puffy white cloud in a blue sky. There she could mentally relax and float, far from pain. This approach got her through her shopping and home again.

Ken, who suffers with rheumatoid arthritis, chooses imagery as a diversion to "take a vacation" from his pain. He sits in his chair, surrounded by the comfort items of a vast music center and many books. If he's reading, which is a way of diverting his attention, he may stop at some point and fantasize about the next portion of the story. Ken has also created a "Fantasy Farm" in his head, where he is the master technician of all that grows in special temperature-controlled buildings. Ken fantasizes about growing perfect apricots in winter, and many other delicacies in this magical place. Ken copes with pain by diverting his attention. He creates a mental environment of perfection.

Barbara, who also suffers from chronic muscle pain, uses imagery as one of many skills to cope with it. Over time, she has developed pain reduction skills that she uses during long work days and while she travels cross country on her job. As she moved from the acute phase of her condition into a chronic one, Barbara also learned the skills of bio-feedback, deep relaxation, meditation, and imagery. She allots one hour in the middle of the day to do these exercises even if it means lying on the floor of a plane flying across the mid-West, or closing the door of her office to practice her pain reducing skills. She isn't secretive or embarrassed about her health needs. Rather than locking herself in isolation, she chooses to share her strategies, and finds affiliation with colleagues who have discovered their own ways to meditate. Intervening early in the cycle of fear-pain-isolation-depression, she takes control by having a plan.

Pain Investigation

An approach that works especially well when pain is intense involves investigating it. This means opening yourself to the pain, leaning into it, softening around it, and allowing yourself to move beyond the anticipated fearful experience. This approach, too, involves using your creative imagination. Stephen Levine writes about this approach in *Who Dies? An Investigation of Conscious Living and Conscious Dying*. He has worked extensively with cancer patients and with others in deep grief. The book includes a helpful section on "Pain Meditations."

Sense of Humor

A sense of humor can also serve as an antidote to suffering. Arthur Schopenhauer, the German philosopher, describes humor as the only divine quality of man. The word humor derives from the Latin, "umor," meaning fluid, liquid--something that flows. Laughter, that spontaneous, irrepressible response to humor, does flow. Laughter can shatter pretensions, bestow humility, restore a sense of balance, strengthen compassion, and bring you to an inner "comfort zone." In addition, when you can laugh at yourself, you are reflecting your sense of transcendence. You are saying, "I--my identity--is separate from this event."

Music

People seem to know intuitively that music heals. This wisdom was incorporated in the ancient healing arts of the Egyptians, Greeks, and during the Renaissance, when a knowledge of music was required of doctors. You can activate your own inner healer by either matching your present mood to a piece of music, or by countering that mood. Ken's wife, Maggie, says she can tell what his pain level is by what music he is listening to. Somber tones tell her he is depressed and wants to be left alone; jazzy ones that he feels better. Music has become a non-verbal way for this couple to communicate. If music is of particular interest to you, develop a plan or consult a music therapist who can devise an individualized program that will help you counter pain.

Self-knowledge

Discover what works for you. Become a part of your treatment team. Resources can be found in the spiritual teachings of Judaism, Christianity, and Eastern philosophies. New Age approaches and scientific investigation are other sources of ideas. You can learn from contemporaries such as Norman Cousins, who emphasized the importance of humor in his chronicle of his experience with ankylosing spondylitis in *Anatomy of an Illness*.[2] He challenges the statistics that say you can't be better than you are, or feel better than you do. While ill he watched old movie comedies and felt better as a result. You can also learn from the two young women whose profiles follow. They both contend with the debilitating fatigue and emotional pain a restricted life imposes upon them and their families.

Gisela and Sheila: Thriving in Their Thirties--Almost

Gisela and Sheila have a great deal in common: both are attractive young married women in their early thirties; sitting side by side they look healthy, even athletic--as if they could be on their way to aerobics class. These women are highly intelligent and well educated; both work in a medical setting; and have symptoms of what is now being called chronic fatigue syndrome (CFS), also referred to as chronic fatigue immune dysfunction (CFID).

Three years ago both were diagnosed as having Epstein-Barr Virus (EBV). This virus is now thought to be relatively rare, and symptoms such as theirs are more often being diagnosed as chronic fatigue syndrome. This syndrome is often experienced by young women who describe exhaustion, difficulty concentrating, headaches, insomnia, and muscle and joint aches. In the recent past, no physical cause could be found for these symptoms. Then came a time of mis-diagnosis, for it resembled not only EBV, but also lupus and fibromyalgia, both chronic illnesses. It sometimes followed mononucleosis, or other viral infections. People like Gisela, Sheila, and the medical profession were perplexed. Recently, Dr. Peter Gott, who writes for Newspaper Enterprise Association, offered hope for the pain and confusion caused by a slippery diagnosis. He wrote that the Center for Disease Control in Atlanta, Georgia, has launched two new studies to define this syndrome, searching for a biomedical explanation for what appears to be undefined malfunction of the immune system. Sheila and Gisela are experiencing the emotional, mental, and social pain that other chronic illness sufferers experience when symptoms and diseases are little understood.

Both women share the psychological, social, and personal concerns common to CFS survivors, but each responds in her own individual way. Sheila has learned to distinguish between the CFS flu symptoms and actual flu virus symptoms and can now better predict the course of her illness. She knows she can lick "regular" flu in a week or less but that the CFS, which she calls "the chronic cruds," will take at least a week's recuperation and sometimes months. Knowing the pattern has helped rid her of some of the guilt for not being able to work.

She says, "I get fatigued profoundly in a way that cannot be warded off; a muscle fatigue where I can't work up enough energy to get out of bed and take a shower. I can't even wash my hair since I don't have the energy to raise my arms. The joint and muscle pains come and go, as do the low grade fevers. When I have a flare-up there can be stabbing pains in the soft muscle tissue. It's all so debilitating. Then out of the blue, I can have ten good days. It would be easier if it made any sense."

Attitudes

Sheila gives herself permission to express her anger while Gisela prefers to leave some things alone. Yet they both cultivate a positive and hopeful outlook.

Therapy

Sheila has benefited from individual psychotherapy but doesn't want to join a support group. Gisela leads support groups but has not sought out therapy for herself.

Fears

Neither of them looks overweight, but they have a constant battle with weight gain due to forced inactivity. A bigger fear they share is that of being around acutely sick people. Gisela is terrified of getting a sore throat and during severe symptoms wouldn't go into the rooms of certain patients in the hospital.

They also have a fear of stress. Both were able to handle an inordinate amount--the kind of pressure that I.C.U.'s and Emergency Rooms generate. "Any stress now makes me non-functional," says Sheila.

Because stress exacerbates CFS, sometimes these young women think that others feel that if they could handle stress better, they wouldn't get sick. There is the subtle implication that a lot of this problem is in their heads. Chronic fatigue syndrome continues to be misdiagnosed as psychosomatic illness or hypochondria. So there is not only the fear of stress, but also the fear of being viewed as neurotic. That kind of innuendo still hurts their feelings.

Support

Sheila and Gisela also say that they suffer from a general lack of true understanding and support. When Sheila was diagnosed as having Epstein-Barr, she found no information in the library or in her nursing books. No one understood or was supportive of her except her doctor. Both women also tire of people saying, "Well, are you exercising?" when they can hardly move.

They found it difficult to get support even among medical people. However, supportive individuals do stand out. The fact that some people view CFS as a fad, "the Yuppie Disease," again, makes them feel "neurotic." In addition, since CFS is sporadic and does not have visible symptoms such as a limp or a rash, sufferers sometimes lose potential support.

Any chronic illness is difficult to deal with, but when a disease is not well accepted or understood by the medical community and the public, the stresses are increased. It is quite common for CFS patients, who wish to maintain their dignity and to think positively, to go out of their way to wear make-up, look well-groomed, and not complain about what they're enduring. Rather than viewing this as a positive step, families, friends and doctors comment that the patient "looks too good to be sick." Health insurance companies are beginning to reimburse for medical expenses related to the diagnosis and treatment of this condition. But there is a lag in its being accepted as a bona fide illness for purposes of reimbursement. This lag can cause the mental and financial anguish of a second victimization.

Career

Both Sheila and Gisela have made many adjustments in their career paths as well. Sheila, an R. N., developed such a fear of picking up another virus on top of the pernicious one that she already has, that she changed the focus of her career. She left "hands on" nursing to go into quality control even though she admits she misses bedside nursing. She has also thought about how she can continue to help people, even if not as a nurse. Once when she gave up her place in line at the supermarket to an old lady, she realized that there really are a lot of different ways to help people if you challenge yourself to find them.

Gisela loves her work. She has severe menstrual pain, due to endometriosis, which is also chronic, but can usually function on pain medication. She feels that she is moving right along, that she is spacing out her long-term career goals. She attributes this partly to finances, and partly to her having less energy. She doesn't push herself as much as she might if she hadn't been ill. She says, "Life is always moving, there is always change, and I am where I am to be. I have learned to enjoy the here and now."

Marriage

The impact of their illness has affected their marriages, too. Both Sheila and Gisela met their husbands-to-be when they were first getting sick. Sheila says, "We certainly had difficulties during our first year. He was going to marry the young, vibrant, busy, work-full-time, clean-the-house, cook-the-supper, socialize, party-with-friends lady. But I'm no longer that person. I used to run at one hundred and ten per cent, now on good days I'm at about seventy five per cent. Maybe I'm a better self. I don't know. I don't know whether I like this self better or not."

Sheila has reprioritized. She saves her energy for part time work, to be with her husband, and to maintain friendships, not for cooking and cleaning. She and her husband have been angry at having to change their life-style.

"It reaches a point when you feel you've got to take control. I got sick and tired of being sick and tired," she says.

Gisela, too, is a different person. She was athletic, was involved in a lot of sports, went swimming for an hour almost every day after a full day of work. She sees people on bicycles and thinks that she should be in their place. But she has to limit what she does.

Gisela and her husband had just met when she began to get sick all the time. "He's Dutch, and with him you work hard and don't complain." It was particularly difficult for them because they were living on a farm where they worked for their room and board. The expectations were high and she couldn't live up to them. "I think that I was kind of an embarrassment to him. I think he thought I was being lazy." After three years of symptoms Gisela now feels much better. This couple has come a long way--he has become more understanding and she has learned to "lighten up" and to be selective about what is important.

Richard, Sheila's husband, has read some books and understands her illness better, too. But, she says, sometimes he forgets, and she tries to leave room for that. And sometimes he just gets tired of it and becomes visibly frustrated.

Personality

Both of these young women have felt changes in themselves as a result of their illness, not only in becoming less physically vigorous, but in their personalities as well. Sheila says, "I am not myself. I'm not what I used to be."

Sheila feels that therapy has helped her, especially in reducing stress. Having been through so much has also enhanced her capacity for empathy and increased her tolerance for "whiners" and "complainers." Now she sees that behavior as a natural stage that most people go through. She's been there. Before she was aware of the patterns, and before she developed coping skills, she complained about how tired she was all the time.

Sheila feels the symptoms and the fears of chronic illness every day, and every day makes decisions that will help her balance her life.

Gisela has developed an interest in herbs and homeopathic medicine and uses this to gain a sense of control and a feeling that she is taking part in the process of healing her endometriosis. She keeps a journal and has learned to be more assertive, especially in setting limits. She feels much better overall and can do more.

Her husband no longer calls her "lazy" and she is less fearful and more hopeful. She feels that, at least for now, she's reached a sense of peace where she is.

Both women have felt deprived of much of the carefree, spontaneous, physical abandon of their age group. It's as if they are maturing early, are developing self-awareness, insight, and tolerance at a more rapid rate than they would if they were not ill.

Sheila and Gisela are being forced to modify their personalities and their life styles, but each is also discovering inner resources she didn't know she had.

Whatever your chronic condition, there is pain and fatigue to contend with. When you can take charge of managing your pain, whether it is more physical or mental, social or emotional, you will perceive yourself as less a victim, and more as a survivor. You will identify less with your disease and more with the positive aspects of your life.

STEPS YOU CAN TAKE TO COPE WITH PAIN AND FATIGUE:

- Consider whether your pain is more physical, mental, emotional, social, or spiritual.

- Review the Pain--Depression Cycle and identify where you tend to get "stuck." Assess where and how you can intervene to improve the quality of your life.

- Begin to develop a library of articles and books that you can tap for a plan of action. Attend classes and workshops.

- Incorporate humor and the release of laughter into your life. Rent videos, attend comedies, follow your favorite cartoonist. And be ever ready to laugh at yourself.

- Learn more about a coping strategy that appeals to you: imagery, music, bio-feedback, or meditation. Develop a plan for applying it.

- Incorporate both medical treatment and mental strategies into your total pain management plan thereby giving yourself (and your doctor) the power and responsibility to make effective therapeutic interventions.

NOTES

5

UNDERSTANDING YOUR FAMILY

Chronic illness demands so much of your attention it is difficult to think beyond it, to be fully aware of the impact of your illness on the family. You know they are suffering, too, but to go through your own grieving process and, at the same time, to assess the changes that are going on within the fabric of your family life can be overwhelming tasks. This chapter addresses the losses and the role changes you and your family face as you begin to adjust to cycles of disabling illness.

Losses

Following is a list of losses to help you determine which apply to you, both individually and as a family, and to what extent. Use this list as a subject for conversation as you and your family begin the process of coping, healing and transcending these losses. Thinking and talking about this may touch off some initial sadness, but remember that grief is only the first step in a process which can end in transcendence and renewed strength.

LOSSES

Physical function
Energy
Sense of control
Independence
Resilience
Patience
Innocence
Security
Competence
Visibility
Privacy
Body-Image
Self-Image
Faith
Expectations for the future
Social contact
Shared responsibilities
Financial power
Self-Esteem
Affection
Autonomy
Optimism
Ability to protect
Sexual communication
Freedom
Equality

Although grief is a universal experience, when you suffer any loss, it is also highly individual. Its uniqueness is partly determined by one's position in the family. The particular ways in which family members suffer survivor-guilt and feelings of helplessness vary according to their age and family role. To complicate matters even more, losses force role-changes, such as from social butterfly to shut-in, from homemaker-volunteer to breadwinner, from authority figure to disempowered dependent, from carefree student to responsible household helper. Such shifts often lead to confusion. Family members wonder who they can rely on for what. Following is a list of possible familial roles. Who, if anyone, assumed these roles before you contracted your illness? What role changes have occurred since then?

FAMILY ROLES

Disciplinarian
Breadwinner
Financial decision-maker
Instructor
Doctor/nurse/veterinarian
Gardener
Cook
Liaison with school
Homework supervisor
Confidant
Rescuer
Nurturer
Victim
Martyr
Handyman
Link to extended family
Social director
Pusher for church attendance
Assigner of household chores
Scapegoat

Changes in roles also affect the equilibrium that served to meet the needs of the various family members. Relationships have to undergo changes to reach a new equilibrium in which as many needs as possible can be met. The high incidence of illness among family members of chronically ill people is an indication of how important it is to understand the dynamics that operate in your family system. Not enough research has been done to draw extensive conclusions about why family members of people with chronic illnesses are so vulnerable to disease. Experience suggests that causes may include simple exhaustion from caring for the ill person, competition for attention and sympathy from the medical team or relatives, over-identification with the ill family member, or a literal attempt to take on his or her pain. These suggestions show how important it is to be aware of your family's reactions and for all of you to develop self-care skills. How each family member handles new roles, anxiety, and depression has direct and indirect bearing on your condition, just as your reactions to your situation has significant impact on theirs.

Emotions of Couples

Subtle myths about family relationships imply that illness brings families together in loving closeness and joy. These myths ignore the power struggles, the double messages that are issued back and forth such as the ill spouse communicating, "Take care of me, but don't encroach on my independence," or the well spouse saying, in effect, "I feel so helpless. I over-control to compensate." Hidden agendas often involve unconscious needs such as the need to keep the ill family member dependent, or to make some member of the family a scapegoat. Martyrdom can mask a need for attention, and authoritarianism can mask in-securities.

As a couple who vowed to be together in sickness and in health, your relationship increases in complexity if one of you is able-bodied and one of you is not. As you move out of the initial crisis stages and begin to adjust to cycles of disabling illness and remission, or as your disease slowly progresses, more time and energy are available to contemplate and make adjustments to your future. Sometimes people think and feel similar things, but they experience their lives differently. They ask different questions. You, the ill spouse may ask, "What will happen to me?" while your well partner's silent query is, "Why did you get sick?"

If you are like most people with chronic illness, you suffer from feelings of helplessness. Because of these feelings you also feel guilty and angry. Your spouse, feeling hopeless and helpless, vacillates between concern and blame. These intense feelings, in turn, cause more guilt and anxiety, and bring on fight/flight responses. After all, who, in their wildest dreams, would have invited disease to the wedding feast?

Maggie Strong, in her book *Mainstay*[1] says, "To become chronically ill is to lose yourself as a healthy person; you grieve. To be married to someone ill and to watch a man or woman you love suffer means you mourn."

How do you and your spouse let go of your expectations of a future in which ill-health had no place? How do you mourn the losses you both see daily, etched in your loved one's face? Dreams about children, career goals, retirement, travel--how can these losses be shared without damaging your relationship? If you and your partner can get in touch with where you are in your own grief cycle, and find a way to go beyond your individual pain to be mutually supportive through sadness and depression, you will go on to restoration--of yourselves individually and as a couple. A couple's cycle of grief looks something like this:

A COUPLE'S GRIEF CYCLE

ILL PERSON	WELL SPOUSE
Denial	
Maybe If I don't give in to my fatigue, it will go away.	I don't want to believe this is happening. Maybe in three months she'll be her old self.
Protest	
I feel betrayed by my own body. Where is God?	Damn it all! This shouldn't be happening to me, to us.

Some days I feel guilty that I'm burdening my family by being sick.

How can I enjoy a good run when he can barely walk? First I feel guilty, then outraged!

Fear

Fear, that't what I feel. What will happen to me in my old age?

The cold jaws of fear tell me that I am alone and responsible for the major efforts for this family. And it will go on and on.

It scares me when I find myself thinking about how they would be better off without me.

Some days I have a fantasy of just walking away from all this, starting out new somewhere. First I feel free. Then the guilt comes crashing down.

It's embarrassing to feel and look so much older than I am.

Where do we belong? Most of our friends have gone away. My partner seems so old. How old am I?

Ambivalence/Bargaining

Just let me get these kids raised before I get much worse.

Just give us a few more good years. We have so much to do.

Sadness/Depresssion

I think I was coping better before. What's wrong with me?

Sad, just sad. That's how I feel most of the time.

Why get up in the morning? I just want to hide in the warm, safe bed.

I feel old before my time. My parents are dealing with the same things we are.

It's lonely in my safe cocoon yet I don't have the energy to get out.

Beat up and worn down, that's how I feel. Oh, to have time for myself or just to rest!

Restoration

If my body is going to be old, my spirit will be young.

This sure makes you grow up in a hurry. I won't say I'd rather not have learned this way.

I've changed a lot. I'm not sure I like the new me.

I've had to temper my impatience. I feel changed. I can't explain it.

I have so much respect for my husband/wife. I didn't know my partner had such strength.

We're making it. There's a mellowness to us, come before our time.

The last relapse was something else. I hope this remission lasts a long time. There's lots to do!

I'm getting familiar with the cycles now. Trust and faith that we'd get to this point kept me going.

My energy is precious. And so is life!

Time is precious. Let's make the most of it.

You may no longer feel equal since your partner can walk away from disability and you cannot. The rhythm of life as a couple is disrupted, but it is a false assumption that illness always disrupts sexual communication. People are apt to become inhibited because they don't know what is appropriate, but the ability of physically impaired people to enjoy sex can often be restored. Some couples report that sexual intercourse tends to relieve the pain, that endorphins may be released that ease tension. Others report that as the drive to achieve becomes more relaxed, as they

67

become less interested in performance and more interested in pleasure, there is more closeness--whether it is in the form of tenderness, comfort, or play.

Emotions of Parents of the Chronically ill:

Although your chronically ill child may be an adult, there is always the sense that you can protect him or her from harm. As your child becomes more ill, the loss of your image as a protector can prove to be most difficult to accept. Because disease, disability, and serious threat to life are supposed to come to the older generation first, there is outrage at the injustice, at the fact that the natural order of events has been violated. Questions that may go through your mind are, "Did I set my child up, unknowingly, to develop this? What can I do to atone? Will he or she be angry at me? What will happen to him when I am no longer here? How can I relieve her suffering? What impact will this have on my own life?"

There is also a tendency to want your loved one to adjust the way that you would adjust, whether through conventional medicine, exercise, diet, religious practices, imaging, stoicism, or denial. You can benefit from education as to the nature of your child's physical problem and the rationale for the treatment program. Such knowledge can help to diffuse your anxiety, and, incidentally, prevent any unconscious attempts on your part to sabotage treatment because of lack of understanding.

Emotions of Children with Chronically Ill Parents:

Children who live in a family with a parent who is chronically ill have a different experience than children who do not. Many adults don't realize that children have the same feelings that they do--fear, anger, sadness, depression, guilt, ambivalence, helplessness, and envy of those more fortunate. However, children at different ages have differing abilities to formulate, work with, and communicate their feelings. Additionally, children are particularly vulnerable to some feelings.

Two factors--the developmental stage of a child and the severity of the onset and progression of a parent's illness have a great deal to do with how that child experiences that illness. The family's capabilities to regroup, communicate, and problem-solve are also factors. One additional factor is the reality that some children seem more resourceful and resilient than others, no matter what their environment. The following information provides a format through which you can understand your children, their particular developmental stages, and how to deal most effectively with their needs at each stage.

Preschool to Seven Years Old

To children in this age group, the whole world revolves around them. The world is created in their image, and they think they should have or can do all things. The younger they are, the more they believe this. Then, when a crisis hits the family, when the attention gets focused on someone else, they experience **fear** that their needs won't be met, **helplessness** to do anything about the situation, and **guilt** that they must have caused the problem. Very young children are not capable of denial, so an **angry** response reflects their basic fears. The usual response a child makes is either to act out or to withdraw. They may also revert to more immature behaviors, such as thumb sucking or bed wetting, and there may be abdominal upsets and a change in eating and sleeping habits. These children will not want to be separated from the family.

HOW TO HELP: Provide sustaining comfort and explain in simple yet accurate terms what is happening. Be aware these simple explanations may have to be repeated often to maintain reassurance. Keep things routine and concrete. Include the child as much as possible in the family activities. It is helpful if one stable person can become the "child's advocate" at stressful times, a person whose job it is to attend to the child's needs. Trust in safe people and safe places is vital.

Ages Seven to Eleven

Children of these ages will feel all of the above emotions, and more, but they will be able to articulate their feelings and thoughts to a greater extent. However, they may revert to behaviors that you thought they'd outgrown, for in fear and under stress it is only human to become "as a (frightened) little child."

This is the age of "magical thinking" and skill building. These are the lovers of scary Halloween dress-ups, and good guy/bad guy movies, where Evil can come to get you, and there is a Fairy Godmother or a Superman to come to the rescue. Children in this age group may be very **angry**, which also masks **fear**.

These are also the years when a social context is being formed; peers are important. Children do not want to be different. **Shame** about not being like the other kids will be felt, followed by **envy** of those who are seen as more fortunate. **Jealousy** towards the parent who's getting all of the attention can also develop. What child this age has not at some time said, "I wish you were dead!" Guilt about these thoughts and feelings can follow.

When a parental role model is ill, there may be **ambivalence** toward that parent. The child may be angry and rebellious, or withdrawn, breeding the seeds for chronic childhood **depression**. Beware, also, of the so-called "good child," the "mommy's helper." This child gets lots of strokes and can all too easily be made into a surrogate parent for the other children, thus aborting the good child's childhood.

HOW TO HELP: Straight talk helps to clarify what's going on. Giving the children things to do helps build skills supporting the paramount developmental task of this age. It can be helpful to "give permission" to the child to feel some of his powerful feelings (anger, embarrassment) by saying something like, "If I were you I'd feel..." Include them in the family, yet be aware of the delicate balance in developing responsibility within a child, yet not asking too much. If the same sex parent is ill (for example, the mother), it is important that the little girl not be thrust into the role of Daddy's mate by letting her assume too many "wifely" chores.

Teens: Twelve to Eighteen

These are the years when the powerful impulses to become self-sufficient are the driving forces of growth. Peers are often more influential than family. There is built-in ambivalence; "I want to go/I want to stay." For teens it is particularly difficult to see their role model ill. Teens do not want to be different, and so they may be embarrassed to be seen with a parent who is not physically fit. Maggie Strong, in her book, *Mainstay,* chronicles painfully and honestly her children's discomfort over their father's illness of multiple sclerosis and the visible deterioration of his mobility. It is confusing to be outraged at parents who are doing their best while at the same time experiencing the thrust for separation and independence which brings about powerful emotions directed at creating the chasm in which leave-taking can occur. For the parent it can be tempting to either push the teenagers out prematurely, or to pull them back into caretaker roles. The teenagers' **fear** causes them to wonder, "Will I, too, someday, be like my parent?" Their **anger** says, "Why can't we be like other families?" Their **embarrassment** whispers, "I don't want to be with you when I'm with my friends."

HOW TO HELP: Provide as normal a teen experience as is possible. Talk with your teen. Encourage a relationship of confidence with another adult, such as a peer's parent, a teacher, or a minister, priest, or rabbi. Don't protect your child from the real you, pain and all. But be careful not to make them feel responsible for making you unhappy.

Children of ill parents can feel older and more mature than their peers. They know first-hand of real, pervasive sorrow. They learn early in their lives that all the love in the world is no protection against pain. They also experience vulnerability early on. One secret fear is that something will happen to the well parent and that no one will be left to care for them. This may not be articulated but will surface when the well parent has a minor illness or needs to go away for a short while. An inordinately strong fear can grip a tiny heart and ask, "What's happening to you? What will happen to me?"

Children of all ages experience difficult emotions, but on the plus side, it should be noted that among all of these powerful feelings, compassion is a feeling that surfaces in children even as young as eighteen months. This is an extraordinary phenomenon not well understood, but nonetheless observed. Children who suffer have, within themselves, the capacity to care deeply and to act on that caring. The seeds of sorrow, when strewn in a loving, capable family, can sprout into compassionate action, even for the young.

Emotions of Siblings

To be a sibling is to be a peer of the closest kind. One's trust and faith in a safe world is shaken when your brother or sister contracts a serious illness. There can be jealousy of the attention and concern that is lavished on the ill sibling. Questions and strong emotions abound. "Will I develop this, too? Why is he or she unlucky, and why am I lucky? What did our parents have to do with this? Will it happen to another of us? What can I do, or should I do, to help? Will I be responsible later? To what extent can I plan my life? Should I have children?"

Since many chronic illnesses have genetic predispositions, each well brother or sister carries "survivor-guilt," coupled with the fear that their own survival is not assured. A combination as powerful as this requires support both within the family and without. Skills are needed to get through the hard times and also to help a family lighten up so that they don't become totally problem-focused.

Emotions of Friends

One woman in her eighties remarked that of all the losses of loved ones, among the hardest for her were not the loss of parents and siblings, but of close friends. For her, friends were her contemporaries, her soul mates, her buffers between family and herself, her traveling companions, her mirrors reflecting back how the world saw her. There is a wide range of intimacy between friends from distant or fickle to closer than family. Friends are the confidants in elementary school, the bearers of dreams during adolescence, the supports of early adult years, and the carriers of our innermost secrets and disappointments of our older years. If the fabric of friendship has been well woven, friends are also with you through hard times, including illnesses.

When your illness threatens the equality of this relationship, friends wonder how they can help. They wonder if you will still have the energy to be available to them and may question whether they did something wrong or caused you any pain. Because such an illness can happen to a loved one, their own lives may seem less secure. In addition, they have their own grief and other emotions to go through as they come to terms with the illness and struggle toward a redefinition of the friendship, based on the new reality of illness.

Despite these fears and challenges, friends can work together with family to provide relief. Friends are challenged to learn more about your particular disease and about you and the friendship, not to mention learning more about themselves! You and your friends can help each other by expressing your caring, and by really listening and hearing each other.

Affection, Intimacy, and Sexuality: What Now?

If you have coped with chronic illness since childhood, you have probably developed ways to meet your needs for affection and intimacy. You have probably confronted your sense of sexuality. If your chronic condition developed recently, you were used to a certain level of affection and intimacy. You had ways of sharing feelings which included words, touching, and quality time together. You may have children, friends, and a mate with whom you freely shared hugs. You may have a partner with whom you developed good sexual communication.

At the time an illness develops, or with an escalation of symptoms, these familiar interactions are challenged. Your self/body image is changing. You may have less energy with which to give of yourself. You may find it physically painful to be touched. Sexually, your disease may seem like an unwanted intruder.

Does sexual activity play havoc with your metabolism? What about painful joints...spastic movement...paralysis? Does chronic fatigue render you too tired to care? Recognizing that you have a problem and wanting to get back on track with this richness of life, is the first step. There are resources available to you through the organization that supports your struggles with your chronic illness. There are trained counselors who can spend a number of sessions with you on intimacy/sexuality issues. Your "sexual vocabulary" and repertoire of sexual and affectional responses can be redefined.

Your friends and loved ones suffer with these issues also. They may be confused as to how to reach out and communicate. Again, there are resources which include easily readable materials. It takes time, energy, and commitment to yourself and your relationships to sort out these sensitive issues. You will find that devoting thoughtful energy to your needs for affection, intimacy, and sexuality helps counter depression and builds self-esteem.

HOW FAMILIES COPE: PROFILES

In the chapter on **Coping With Pain and Fatigue**, Gisela and Sheila tell of the early days of both their marriages and their adjustments to chronic illness. What follows is the profile of a couple who have coped for over twenty-five years with several chronic conditions.

Ken and Maggie: A Couple that Copes

Their home is spacious with wide doorways that accommodate a wheelchair, and a specially designed chair that tilts forward so Ken can get out of it easily. Outside there is a garden for Maggie.

A picture of a beautiful Korean child in full colorful Korean costume catches your eye, and Ken and Maggie, both talking at once, tell you that she is Toriane, their adopted grandchild. They have two adored granddaughters, McKensie and Toriane, but

Toriane at four years has shown a special sensitivity to her "Opa" and his physical problems. She has learned not to rush up to him no matter how glad she is to see him, because he can be knocked down very easily. She also knows that he's had hand surgery and that his bones hurt. Toriane is gentle with Opa and asks him how his "owies" are. She asks if there are any on his face to be sure it's O.K. to kiss him. She even drew a picture of his pain--a jagged, zig-zagging black line in his bones. This tiny child communicates concern and understanding of his pain.

Ken was diagnosed in 1963 as having rheumatoid arthritis. He had experienced painful swelling of his knees for years prior to his diagnosis. The onset of his disease occurred after a particularly serious strep throat infection. The job stresses as a Utilities Supervisor in the United States Air Force overseas didn't help.

Maggie and Ken had plans. He would retire and they would both go to college, get degrees, join the Peace Corps, and try to be stationed in Turkey, where they had served in their Air Force days.

But chronic illness changed all that. Eventually, Ken retired early; there was a drop in their income with all the accompanying adjustments, and he could no longer get around. Ken has had both knee joints replaced, one of them twice. His right foot has been reconstructed, and he's now having reconstructive surgery on his hand. He did get to college, and it was a help in getting over that "period where every thing was falling apart." The closeness of their family--they have one son, William--helped the most.

Maggie has to take care of everything, and this is frustrating to both of them. When the laundry and cooking and cleaning and marketing are done, she has all of the outside work to do. Ken relates, "She's painted the house, taken care of the car and the yard, front and back, and laid about four tons of flagstone." It makes him angry that he can't help her more. He says she is a good student, that he's even taught her how to do carpentry. Once when she was hammering he said, "Harder!" and she got angry. He said, "Just pretend that that's my face you're hitting on!" and then they both laughed. But she describes those first years as devastating.

Their philosophy of life helped them to cope with the devastation. Ken and Maggie both feel that the time they spent in Turkey had a profound impact on them and that some of the Moslem belief in Kismet--predestination--may have rubbed off on them. "If something is going to happen, it's going to happen," they say.

"Sometimes I feel as if I've lived eight lives," says Maggie. She lived through air raids in Vienna and has been on trains that have been bombed. Sometimes she believes that everything that happens, happens for a reason; that if you hang in there long enough, things will get better.

Recent developments sometimes make it hard to hang on to those beliefs. In November, 1987, Maggie learned that she had breast cancer. She made a remarkable recovery from surgery; she was in the hospital for only two days and was back on her regular work routine in three or four. The drainage bag from the incision got in her way while doing household chores so she found an old fashioned cobbler's apron, ripped out one of the seams to make a larger compartment to accommodate the bag, and wore it inside out. She soon was back to swimming and gardening every day. Maggie believes "God just made us (women) stronger. We have an extra layer of fat."

A few months later, Ken felt a rough spot in his throat. They both laugh as they recount how Maggie was hardly over her surgery before Kenny had to be operated on for cancer of the throat. Undergoing nine weeks of radiation resulted in his teeth being destroyed, and the loss of his sense of taste. For Kenny, this has been a big loss. He misses sweets, especially since his wife bakes wonderful Viennese pastries. Recently, though, he's been able to again taste sage, green pepper, cinnamon and strawberries.

Ken enjoys his visits to the V.A. Hospital because he belongs to a group that has been used to test experimental medications for several years. He and his cronies there are known for their "gallows humor," and Ken knows that the humor and the camaraderie help.

Ken volunteers for the Arthritis Foundation and goes to the Easter Seal heated swimming pool three times a week where he is a favorite "caller" for the exercise instructions. He seems to start informal support groups of one kind or another wherever he goes. One such group consists of several couples who get together every Sunday morning for conversation and a walk on the beach. Ken goes along on his scooter, or sits in the car and listens to jazz until the others get back from their stroll.

Maggie copes on a high level, too. She swims every day, gardens, and walks. She likes to walk alone. "You can think and get ideas about how to get around the bad times. It's also a time to pray," she says. Maggie thinks you learn a lot from having been down. She's learned to listen to her body and to take better care of herself. She's less of a perfectionist about her housework, and sometimes she'll stay in bed in the morning until eight o'clock instead of seven fifteen.

They have their separate ways of coping which balance all they do together. Sometimes they wonder how they have lived through so much and speculate that the body is very resilient. But Ken and Maggie are resilient in more ways than one, having learned to be content with little things. Their mutual support is obvious; he's enthusiastic about how helpful she is to the veterans at the hospital; she's outspoken in her praise of his sense of humor. He speaks lovingly of how he found her in Vienna and of how she couldn't speak English. She comments on the large number of wives who leave their husbands after a diagnosis of rheumatoid arthritis, and of how glad she is that she didn't do that.

Among the many pleasures they share is music. As mentioned in the chapter on pain, Maggie can read Ken's mood from the kind of music he chooses to listen to. Wagner indicates depression, while waltzes and jazz mean his spirits are up again.

The mutuality in all of these experiences represents an emotional investment in a shared history. This investment is now paying off in the strength, perseverance, and courage they are able to bring to the crises in their lives as individuals and as a couple. They have learned much about themselves and each other, and through investing in their family, they have found much to value and to love.

Jeanne Naspo: Post Poster-Child

Jeanne Naspo and her family developed coping skills when she was growing up with a rheumatic disease which began in her infancy. Have you ever wondered what happens to poster children after they grow up? What follows the publicity and fanfare? Jeanne Naspo, the first poster child for the Arthritis Foundation thirty years ago, toured the White House with Mamie Eisenhower and was interviewed by Mike Wallace. Now, thirty years later, she is a successful family counselor. She uses crutches after having had four joint replacements (both hips and both knees) and weighs only 57 pounds--57 pounds of determination to be as independent as possible, and to enjoy life. Her tiny frame is barely four feet nine inches tall, with delicate arms and hands that are permanently knotted up almost into fists, but when she takes your hand in both of hers you feel connected to her through her warm, large hazel eyes. You immediately feel comfortable. This small vibrant person works forty hours a week as a Vocational Counselor for the state and is developing a private practice in family counseling with special consideration given to those of any age who are dealing with major/chronic illnesses.

Jeanne has given much thought to the impact serious illness has on the family, as well as on the individual. She believes that one reason she is successful is that her parents did not treat her like a **sick** child. Jeanne developed juvenile rheumatoid arthritis when she was eight months old, but it wasn't diagnosed until she was two and a half.

Jeanne describes her mother and father as bright, level-headed and supportive parents. She says, "If it weren't for my mother's loving care I'd be a bitter person. She is a wonderful role model, too." Her mother developed lupus at age 37, and is now on dialysis.

"As for my dad, he taught me a lot about having fun. He would sit with me when I couldn't walk and practice his music. He'd play the saxophone to Frank Sinatra records. I learned all of the words to all those songs." The Greeks believed that music restored health to both body and soul; perhaps Mr. Naspo's nurturing is another reason Jeanne isn't bitter.

But Jeanne is also well aware of the impact that illness can have on siblings. Her sister, Joan, who is two-and-a-half years younger, does not always seem to have as much self-confidence as Jeanne has. As Jeanne puts it, "Joan was faced with having to accept not only my physical limitations, but all of the extra attention I was given as well." Most family problems are compounded by the presence of physical disability, and sibling rivalry is no exception.

Families tend to take great care of the sick child. "There was emphasis on my becoming educated, on planning ahead for me so I would be able to take care of myself, while it was taken for granted that my sister would get married, that she would be able to take care of herself. I was praised often for things I did. I didn't stand up until I was five years old. Everything I did, I was encouraged."

Jeanne believes reinforcement and encouragement do work to build confidence and self-esteem, but she also believes there has to be something from within, too. Despite all that encouragement, Jeanne felt a need to prove herself. "I wanted so much to be independent!" she says. If there is not that basic desire to do well, if there isn't that inborn drive, no amount of outside encouragement will work. She sees evidence of this in her clients. As long as there is that struggle to come to terms with a problem, counseling can help.

Until recently there has been little education in how to come to terms with the feelings that are aroused in the ill person and in the family when a chronic disease occurs. For example, Jeanne didn't deal with her feelings as a child. "I did what my mother and the doctors told me. I went to physical therapy, did my assigned chores, but I didn't confront and deal with the pain until much later."

After she completed her Master's degree at 27 and was ready to start her career, she had a flare-up of her illness, which brought her plans to a standstill. She went through a bad time. It was then that she made the heavy decision to have the joint replacements. At that time she had been in a wheel chair for about two years and was suffering severe and almost constant pain. Her goal was to get it all over with as quickly as possible so that she could get to work. When the pain and some of the restrictions were gone, she "felt like a free woman, that the world was out there for me, that there wasn't anything I couldn't do." Her eyes sparkle as she recalls her joy at being physically fit enough to sit behind a desk, to walk out of her office to the reception area--albeit with crutches--to be out among people, to get a salary and to be able to set new goals.

"It was a treat to be able to stand up and do my own dishes. The more responsibility I was given, the more I ate it up," she says. Jeanne has a lot of insight about how she handles that struggle between dependence and independence that goes along with chronic illness and is so much a part of travelling toward transcendence. "People tell me that I have accepted my disability so well and that I have made such a good 'adjustment.' They talk as if you go to a certain point, and then you're 'adjusted.' I have to make adjustments every day. It's an ongoing process. You don't reach a certain age, then get adjusted and live happily ever after. Your life changes daily." An example of such a decision is whether to dress herself, which takes almost three hours, or to hire an attendant to help her to dress and use the saved time for professional pursuits.

Along with these decisions, there are constant role changes. She has to hire a driver because she cannot drive a car, and she has to have an attendant wash her hair because she cannot raise her arms above shoulder height. Then she goes to work and leaves this highly dependent role behind as she shifts to her role as a highly independent, competent career woman seeing disabled people for vocational rehabilitation and private clients for family therapy. "I have a hundred responsible decisions to make so it's back and forth, and back and forth, every day." These shifts from being cared for to caring for herself and others mean a life of constant readjusting.

Constantly readjusting is exhausting and it is difficult to work around the fatigue. "My fear is that I might give in to it, get too comfortable being a couch potato," she says. This seems unlikely. For example, when she was isolated because of her illness, she would do **anything** to keep herself sane, to stay stimulated mentally. "I would set up projects--whatever I could do, I would do." She will always be a goal-setter, but that involves constant readjustment to different levels of fatigue, flares, and remissions, along with the usual demands that face anyone with a full-time job and a private practice as well.

Jeanne knows that sometimes she does too much. She attributes this to an underlying fear that she won't be able to sustain her current level of energy. She acknowledges, too, that if a disabled person calls in sick it is apt to be assumed that the job is too much for him or her because of the disability.

Jeanne is quick to accept the gains that she has made as a result of being disabled, the patience that she has learned and the appreciation of little things. She enjoys what she does. Her statement, "I get **so** much enjoyment out of life!" is totally convincing. She also has become disciplined and feels that she has developed a good sense of perspective.

When asked what advice she has for people with chronic illness, she replies, "Respect the pain. When you are diagnosed as having a chronic disease you need to educate yourself about it. Know your disease and take responsibility for the management of it. Get practical guidelines for living with it and working around your fatigue level."

She also makes a strong point of spending time to become more introspective. This is an important step in learning to deal with your frustrations. "Have goals," she adds. "This is especially important after the diagnosis. When one can't see past the illness -- that's sad. I enjoy going to wherever I'm going."

Jeanne sees many people with mental and emotional handicaps and she says she would so much rather have a physical one. Of course some people become emotionally impaired as a result of a physical disability but then, says Jeanne, you often don't know which came first. She affirms herself with, "I am not a disabled person mentally," and "I am strong and independent emotionally." She not only is, but she is helping a lot of other people to be emotionally strong and independent, too.

Summary

As couples, as family, as friends, attentive listening is a gift you can give to each other. If these intense emotions that you and your loved ones feel are reflected back, you and they feel validated. Progress toward spiraling upward spiritually, though you may be spiraling downward physically, is facilitated.

Your manner of coping is, of course, highly individual, but if you and your loved ones find it difficult to communicate your feelings and make these changes in roles on your own, help is available. Support groups can meet many such needs of family members. A support group is necessary if you don't have people you can talk to on a confidential basis, feeling free to express some of your negative emotions. Family, marital and individual therapy are also viable options to consider.

If you can keep communication open among members of your family, adjust to new roles with flexibility, develop higher level self-care skills, and examine and work through your own attitudes, then you and they will grow through the experience and will become closer. Over time, after you have identified and mourned the losses and role changes, you will be able to let go of the old expectations and goals and find new ones. As with Ken, Maggie, and Jeanne, with the courage and the clarity that seem to be a gift of suffering, it is possible to find a way to inject a new quality into your family life that none of you has known before. The chapter that follows, **Learning Together; A Matter of Heart**, illustrates how one family developed skills, found support, and now transcends the frustrations and fears of chronic illness.

NOTES

6

LEARNING TOGETHER: A MATTER OF HEART

When one person in a family has a chronic illness, emotions and experiences of all the members are colored by the knowledge that the ill person is struggling. It means that **all** members of the family are struggling, each in his own way. This chapter is written by the wife of a man with a chronic heart disease because the focus is on the family rather than on the chronically ill person.

The specifics of this family's experience may differ from those of others, but their struggle will be recognized by families where there is a member with a chronic illness, whether it be a heart problem or some other ongoing disease. Greta tells how she grew through her struggle in her own way.

Greta's Story

My husband first learned he had heart disease about 10 years ago when he was 37 years old. Later we learned that unlike many heart conditions, his is a chronic illness. Our lives, our children's lives, our marriage, have certainly been changed because of this, but they have not been dominated by it. There's still a lot of laughter and closeness in our home. We all seem to enjoy one another and seldom tire of being together or talking with each other. The kids still love to bring their friends over and include them, for a while, into our family.

But it has been a struggle. For one thing, we each have our own distinct way of handling information, whether it's negative or positive. Generally, my husband, John, seems to cope best through letting news sink in and then "forgetting" it. He has a unique capacity (one which I've envied at times) of being up-beat and humorous on almost any occasion, but it's not the kind of optimism that's Pollyanna-ish and hollow. He seems to be a genuinely happy person, despite the circumstances, and has made me aware, time and again, that laughter is often the best medicine.

I, on the other hand, tend to take things more seriously, to think about them until I've settled them in my mind and my heart. I'm not a worrier; I just know that, for me, I have to face pain as it comes, deal with it, and then go on.

Our younger son, now 14, is more like me. He takes things to heart, too, only he says what he's thinking, and in a more blunt way. That's good for our family; we sometimes need someone to start us talking. Our older son, too, is extremely sensitive, but, like his dad, tends to keep his thoughts and feelings to himself. More than once, his steadiness and soft-heartedness have been invaluable to me.

I make such a point of our reactions because one of the tasks which is crucial if a family is to transcend chronic illness is the recognition and acceptance of the fact that each person does, almost automatically, react differently. For me, accepting this fact was quite difficult. If I were sad, for instance, I wanted someone to be sad with me, and, on the occasions when John seemed to be too glib about a situation which I considered crucial, I'd get depressed and resentful. It took me a long time to respect and value his way of dealing with things as uniquely his and to stop trying to change him into a clone of me. And, I have to confess, we sometimes still have trouble talking about our fears. I need consolation, and John needs me to drop the subject. It's a dilemma.

This is only one of the hurdles we've had to surmount. For example, one of the obstacles I've wrestled with this year is the feeling of being liberated into middle age, ready to enjoy my career and my life, and yet sensing, sometimes, that, in many ways, John has been prematurely catapulted into old age. I'm ready to plan a skiing trip, and he's on the couch napping. Or we set out to enjoy the day and return two hours later because he doesn't feel well.

Such daily surprises and adjustments are difficult to live with without feeling concerned, resentful, and then guilty. However, the fact that the feelings I have (that we all have) are normal is a big comfort to me. I cope by letting myself feel them, telling myself it's okay to feel them, sharing them with John or not, depending on whether it's necessary, and then substituting some activity we can both enjoy. However, this coping has been hard-won and still is difficult to implement at some times, and impossible at others.

It's true, I think, that any crisis challenges peoples' equilibrium and forces them to re-think almost everything, and chronic illness is nothing if not an on-going crisis. The unique form it takes, though, (depending on the illness), is that it's often like an accident waiting to happen. Just when one feels lulled into a sense of life's normalcy, something occurs which begins the process of readjustment all over again.

Perhaps this is more true of heart disease than of some other chronic illnesses. The pattern for us, at least until recently, has been of fairly long asymptomatic periods interrupted by sudden, unexpected crises. One's adrenal system never quite has permission to fully relax and think, "Whew! That's over for good." Over time, that constant pattern of being almost-on-guard can be quite wearing. It leaves you wide open to the uncontrollable factors in life, and then demands that you find a way to cope with them--if necessary, for the rest of your life.

For us, the first unexpected crisis, of course, was John's diagnosis. Five days later, he underwent double by-pass surgery. I have to admit I was terrified. By-pass surgery, even then, was rather routine, but not for our family. All I knew was that they were going to saw open his breast bone, stop his heart from beating, repair it, and sew him back up. Routine or not, it seemed drastic to me.

Hospital stays are never easy, especially when they occur as abruptly as ours had. One day everything seemed normal, and the next day it felt as if John's life were up for grabs. Suddenly, our whole routine was shattered--the way we thought, the way we planned, the way we slept, even, sometimes, the way we breathed. I knew this was an event that none of us could control and that it was bound to change all of us permanently, and that sense of being hurtled toward an unsolicited turning point was (and still is, at times) horrendously frightening. Having no idea about what the future held, we had no idea if any of us would be able to adapt to it.

Two things really helped me, though: I had a faith in God that kept me believing, all the way through, that both John and I were loved and that we were being well taken care of. Also, I had a truly special group of friends whom I knew would stand by me, no matter what. We were fortunate, too, in that the hospital not only had an outstanding cardiac team, but one which, at that time, provided pre-surgical counseling for patients.

We learned that research suggested that pre-op counseling often helps to lower post-surgical depression. The head cardiac nurse spent a lot of time with us, answering our questions and just letting us get to know and trust her. That, and a few volunteers from Mended Hearts (an association of survivors of by-pass surgeries) helped immensely. We didn't feel quite so alone.

Still, there were nagging concerns. At that time, our sons were 9 and 4, and I had been out of the job market for over three years. I didn't even dare to wonder, if worse came to worst, how I could support them. Instead, I tried to compartmentalize my concerns into "pre-surgery" and "post-surgery" categories, a kind of "Let's get through this first, and then we'll think about what to do next."

But it was a frightening feeling. People always say that when spouses or lovers share problems, they grow closer, but in our marriage that had not been my experience. Both of us had been raised in families where painful emotions were borne silently and in private. In fact, when I was growing up, it was considered ungrateful to be sad or to show sad feelings. Smiling and acting like nothing was wrong meant you were strong. So I'd learned early to hide my sadness, and at the time of the first surgery (ten years ago) I still hadn't unlearned it.

Also, John and I were, and are, very protective of each other. It's difficult to cry over someone's possible incapacity or death when that person is sitting right next to you. The tendency is to cry alone to spare him. Because we had few skills to help us share our fears, each of us tried to convince the other that we weren't at all worried. All we really succeeded in doing, however, was isolating ourselves.

Even so, there were some moments in which the fear and uncertainty broke through to both of us at the same time, and we knew we were alone--John, me, and Fear, locked in a compelling dance, choreographed by strangers. One of those times occurred the night before the surgery. Even though I had planned to stay with him as long as I could, John asked me to leave at about 7 p.m. He was extremely quiet as I prepared to leave, and he hardly reacted as I hugged him good-bye. I made it about halfway down the hall and decided to go back and give him another hug. It was so hard to think of him lying there by himself all night. As I walked in, he took one look at me and started to cry, and then we both cried. He told me later that he'd been convinced that night that he'd never see me or our children again.

Despite our concerns, the surgery went extremely well. Within five weeks, John was back to work full-time, looking tan and healthy and slim. The more he recovered, the more young and vital he looked and acted. Until he resumed normal speed again, neither of us realized just how much he had slowed down. This was one adjustment that was positive and pleasant to make.

The other big change in our life, of course, was his diet. We had been the prototypical meat-and-potatoes family with a fair amount of fast foods thrown in. One of our favorite pastimes had been to go out late at night and have long discussions over fried eggs, ham, and hashbrowns. Lots of memories revolved around this particular coffee shop or that special conversation.

It wasn't just the food which drew us; it was a part of a lifestyle of two young parents who needed some time away and who usually couldn't afford much more than a couple of dollars. This habit, so tied into the fabric of our marriage, was especially hard to break. But break it we did. This set up a pattern which still continues today, a pattern of slowly having to lose parts of our lives that have meant a lot to us.

That litany of loss was to reverberate through the ensuing years, time and time again, and with each loss came, for me, a cycle of denial, anger, depression, bargaining, and finally acceptance-- the same cycle one goes through in mourning a physical death. However, even letting myself admit to having these feelings was a difficult step; it literally took years before I fully believed that it was not inconsiderate to cry or to be angry at a painful situation.

With the type of personality I have, it helped me a lot to finally realize that all those stages were just the emotions' way of reacting to challenging situations and that those emotions were there to help me, not to hinder me. Denial, on the other hand, not only got lonely for me, but it also numbed me out and gave me less of a range of emotions to work with. And I needed all the help I could get.

One other loss we faced was not so easily brushed away. On one of John's early post-op check-ups, his doctor informed us that John had a specific kind of heart disease, one which had a somewhat worse prognosis than we had thought. His body over-produces cholesterol, so in spite of diet and medication, his vascular system would continue to self-obstruct. The real stunner, though, was that this particular strain had a strong genetic component, and that male children, rather than female, were at higher risk to develop it.

"You'd better have your sons' cholesterol checked," the doctor advised. I remember sitting there in the leather chair in his office, quiet, still, almost immobilized with shock.

"Well," I thought, "in the space of one minute you've just wiped out my entire family, everyone I love."

This new threat meant that not only might we lose our present way of life, but also our potential future, our hopes and our dreams for our sons. This was not the first time, nor would it be the last, that I had the sensation of walking out of a doctor's office feeling as if an emotional bomb had been dropped on us.

We did have the boys tested, and, surprisingly, it was our four-year-old (the seemingly more athletic one with the healthier diet) who tested out as more susceptible than the nine-year-old. Now the whole family began the slow process of changing diets and lifestyles. Emotionally, the only way I could cope with all of this was to focus in on the joys and sorrows of each day as it came and not look any further than sundown for my hope. In fact, I have to say that developing the ability to live in the present has been one of those strange, but welcome, gifts that often turn crises into mixed blessings. It's really been the only sane way for me to handle this.

For the next five years, John's health continued to be good, if not excellent, and it was difficult to know how to feel about his illness. John basically took the stance that he not only was well, he was much better off than most men his age.

I, on the other hand, was leery about feeling that complacent. His dad had had four major heart attacks and several other members of his family had died of heart disease before the age of 45. The disease seemed to surround us, even as we tried to escape it.

Still, I, too, functioned fairly well until our younger son was hospitalized for three and a half months with a potentially threatening illness. This occurred about four years after John's surgery and just ten days after I had had a hysterectomy. John took our child's hospitalization harder than I've ever seen him take anything. In fact, for the first three days, all he did was cry, and the crying jags brought on angina he hadn't felt in years. I wondered, at times, if I were going to lose both of them. It wasn't until ten months later (once I knew our son was out of danger) that all the stress caught up with me--with a vengeance. I had never really taken the time to recover from the hysterectomy, either physically or emotionally, and now I found myself crying at the slightest thing. One day I cried because I couldn't make the bed correctly; the sheet was sticking out from under the bedspread. Most of the time I felt totally inadequate and worthless.

Also, I didn't feel like eating, and my sleep was fitful and irregular. I began to wonder why I was even alive and became convinced that my family and friends would be better off without me. I was sure I was spoiling all my family's happiness by being so unhappy.

After six months or so, my despair became so great that I began to think of ways to kill myself. Why live, I thought, just to see everyone else die? To help me out, my best friend took me, for a week, to her parents' home on a farm. I remember trudging through the muddy fields, hour after hour, begging God to give me one good reason to live. On the trip home, I decided to get some medical help.

Again, this excruciating experience turned out to be, I see now, an impetus for me to grow. The doctor diagnosed a severe depression, put me on anti-depressant medication, and began to teach me how to change my negative thought patterns into more positive ones. He taught me how to see myself and my situation realistically, rather than through the lens of hopelessness and helplessness.

I worked hard at following his suggestions, and gradually, life didn't look quite so black anymore. An added bonus was that these skills of assessing situations realistically would later help me deal with John's disease. Once again, crisis had bred the ability to cope.

I attended Bible studies to try to understand, and I tried harder than ever to build strong and lasting relationships with our sons. I, for example, was the one who taught them to catch, throw and hit. And--this was a biggie for me--I decided, at age 41, to go back to school to acquire some marketable skills.

This last decision was emotionally difficult. I still felt stupid and worthless at times, and I was terrified of failure. More threatening than that though, was the link in my mind between John's illness and my return to school. I remember saying to a friend, "Registering for those classes means I admit that some day John will die." It was hard; I cried on my way to my first class.

During my second year of school, we began to realize again that John's condition was definitely worsening. He began to experience some angina, some shortness of breath. His stamina declined and his naps increased. Over the next year he had several angiograms and was put on an extensive medical regimen--blood thinners; fish oil; aspirin; cholesterol-lowering medications. We laughed about how our lives were beginning to be governed by the little beeper on his pill box, but it was true. However, we kept reminding ourselves how lucky we were to live in an era when so much could be done for cardiac patients and how fortunate we were to have the doctors we had. It really did help to look at what we did have, rather than what was slowly eroding away.

But there came a time, in December of 1986, when an angiogram showed four arteries substantially blocked, two of them being those originally by-passed. They told us they would do a quadruple by-pass this time, and they also cautioned us that each surgical procedure was slightly more risky than the previous one.

The operation was scheduled for six days before Christmas. Our goal was to have him home by Christmas Eve. I, in particular, told myself I didn't care what shape he'd be in when he returned; we just wanted him home for the holidays.

Although the surgery was in the same hospital, with almost all of the same doctors, the hospital experience for us was different this time. John was admitted only one day before the surgery, and, to our disappointment, the counseling and comfort we'd received the first time were lacking. (Those programs had been cut due to more stringent insurance coverage. Most patients were admitted only one day before surgery--hardly enough time for counseling.)

Although the doctors visited as scheduled, we were left alone with our own thoughts and fears and that factor alone made the second surgery much more difficult to bear. To make matters worse, John had found out a day earlier that he had lost his job. Thus, he would be faced with recovering without a job to recover to.

Even more devastating, perhaps, was that, because of pre-existing conditions, we now needed private health insurance. The fees were astronomical! Reluctantly, we decided to just insure John.

Needless to say, everything seemed pretty bleak as we waited for that surgery, but we both kept our senses of humor well-honed for the occasion, and we actually did have a few good laughs that week. Again, living in the present, rather than in the future, helped to lessen the stress. Each night I would thank God for the fact that all four of us had been safe that day, and I would mean it. It was cause for thanksgiving.

John came home on December 23, but it was difficult to drum up much Christmas cheer. I remember in the middle of Christmas Day falling asleep in some old sweatpants and a sweatshirt, only to be awakened by a friend who had dropped by on the way to a party to bring us some homemade pie. I took one look at her in her coordinated Christmas outfit, glanced down at my own sweat-pants, and began to sob. There was a normal life out there somewhere, but we weren't a part of it.

John did not improve as rapidly as he had after the first surgery. Two weeks after it the first crisis came. One midnight, in severe pain, John asked me to call the paramedics. Two scenes from that night remain riveted in my mind: one is the sight of John, whitish-gray, soaked with sweat, gasping for breath, doubled over in pain. The other is the sight of my younger son's face as he watched the paramedics carry his dad out on a stretcher into the ambulance.

As I followed the ambulance to the hospital, I thought about all the other times, late at night, when I had driven this same road with him in the passenger's seat, fearful and in pain, saying, "Hurry! Hurry!"

I also remember thinking, rather too calmly, "Well, I'm glad my sister is here for the holidays. Now I don't have to worry about her arriving in time for the funeral." I was surprised that shock could make me feel so dispassionate.

As it turned out, this episode was one of a series of similar "emergencies" that were to plague us throughout that year. John's recovery continued to be slow; February and March I remember as particularly long months as we began to realize that, even if John did find work, it was questionable as to whether or not he felt strong enough to take it. He applied for and got state disability. That helped.

However, it soon became obvious that we needed more income, so we took out a third mortgage on our home. We had taken the second one out to pay a large hospital bill. Occasionally, as those funds began to dwindle, I would read stories of the newly-homeless, some of whom had lost their homes due to catastrophic illnesses, and think, "That could happen to us." I was torn between staying in school for my last year or giving up that dream to find just any job. I already had the equivalent of two part-time jobs, but they barely made a dent.

Still, we did manage to have some fun, too. Occasionally, we went to the cheaper mid-day movie matinees and joked about being senior citizens before our time. And, whenever I wasn't too swamped with homework, we took walks and browsed around the bookstores. Meanwhile, John was getting stronger, but the bouts of abdominal pain continued.

There was another problem which began to have an almost daily impact on us; our younger son, now 13 and in junior high, was having trouble dealing with the fact that his dad wasn't working when almost everyone else's dad was, and that his dad was not well, either. He got angry, he got surly, and he spent a lot of time complaining and trying to argue with us. Underneath it all, he was scared. I didn't blame him.

One day in the spring, as baseball tryouts approached, he asked me, point blank, "Why can't I have a dad who can practice baseball with me like everybody else's does?" There wasn't a lot I could do for him but listen. I felt the same way myself sometimes. It was sad to see other couples our age playing tennis or hiking. It was time to enjoy life, not restrict it.

Finally, in October, John's abdominal problem was diagnosed as gallstones, and a week later he had his gall bladder removed. For John, this surgery was physically much harder than the other two, and for me, it took quite an emotional toll. I remember making a friend promise that if anything went wrong in this surgery he would put me in a strait jacket in a psychiatric hospital, and I was serious. I knew that I was getting dangerously close to the end of my ability to cope.

Again, the surgery itself went well, but the recovery was painful and slow. However, we were greatly encouraged when a month later, John was offered a full-time job and I a half-time job, just when we'd about depleted our savings.

However, after a few months, we could both see that the three-hour round-trip commute and the stress of the job were taking their toll on John. His color alternated between ashen gray and yellowish-white; his bouts of angina became more frequent. Toward the end of each day, I would run the stairs for him whenever he needed something, and, for the first time in our marriage, I did almost all of the housework without his help. On the one hand, I loved helping him--he'd always been so good about showing gratitude. On the other hand, I was scared. How much worse could this get before we'd have to make drastic changes in our living situation?

Thus, we tenuously began another stage of chronic illness, that stage in which the equal balance between the two partners begins to shift. I was working really hard now, in school full-time, plus three part-time jobs (about an 80-hour week). Still, I wanted to be so careful that John didn't feel as if he weren't pulling his own weight, because he was. Just getting through a work day was a major triumph for him.

In July two turning points occurred. The night our new medical insurance came through, I ended up in the emergency room of the hospital with my own chest pains. John sat in the waiting room with an angina attack, worrying about me. In the end, they diagnosed a minor case of mitral valve prolapse (a non-threatening condition), but the experience gave me great pause; how long could I keep on working so hard?

The second thing that happened was that John had a minor heart attack on the freeway on the way to work. Paramedics got him to the hospital in time and he recuperated quickly and well, but that incident left its mark on me. The threat of something happening on the freeway, which I'd previously ignored, even though he often got angina attacks while driving, had now become a reality. The doctors also told him that there was a substantial chance he would have another minor vessel close up again (another minor heart attack).

That fall was the most difficult time of all. Both of us wrestled, separately and together, with quality-vs-quantity-of-life issues, and about where to go from here. Some new medications were greatly alleviating his angina, but John was still having trouble making it through the workdays, and weekends were mostly spent recuperating.

Finally he decided that to work any longer was to risk some serious consequences. What he wanted was to either get a less stressful job, or, if he couldn't do that, to quit and try to work out of our home. I was relieved and surprised at the same time. For John to quit work at age 46, to give up all of his professional dreams, was a huge step on his part, and an admission, I thought, of just how bad he was feeling.

I was truly moved by his courage and honesty; rather than be the macho man who worked until he dropped, he was being honest with himself and with me. I appreciated that. I knew, above all, I had to be flexible. John wasn't saying, "I want to quit." He was saying, "I have to quit." It felt like do or die.

We spent a couple of months discussing finances, deciding how and if we could swing this, all the while realizing we probably didn't have a choice. One factor, especially, made the decision difficult; with heart disease, and with John's particular medical profile, we were told that his life expectancy ranged anywhere from about one year to twenty. That's quite a range to plan for, financially and emotionally. Of course, we both had feelings of "How can we make it?" Once again, I experienced that strange time warp of just gearing up my own life while living with someone who was "retired."

I also went through a period of mourning for all the things we probably would never have and do if he quit work. For a while, I wasn't sure whether we were giving up on life or opting for it. This time, however, we talked much more openly about all this; the years had taught us something.

We also tried to think of all the positives involved. We'd have more time together, and he'd have more time with the kids. He could help run the household while I worked. We'd changed roles once before, much earlier in our marriage, so knowing that we'd previously handled it well helped.

As of now, it seems we've made a good decision. The most obvious proof is that John's happiness seems to be reflected in generally better health (more stamina, better color, lack of angina). An added bonus has been that his free-lance work has, so far, been in demand, yet he does it at his own pace. And because we've divided the professional and household labor more equally, we both feel like much more of an equal twosome than we have for a long time.

This new stage, however, has brought its own unique problems. Because John's around more, I find myself wondering just how close to him I really want to become. How much intimacy am I willing to risk? I find myself spending more time outside the home, building a career and friendships of my own. I was relieved when I read this was a healthy thing to do.

I've also read that spouses of the chronically ill often feel neither single nor married, at least not in the way they formerly did. For me, that is sometimes true. At times, such ambiguous feelings are truly difficult to deal with.

Still, we continue to look at what we do have. John has been virtually pain free for a few months, our relationships with both our children are excellent, and we have not only survived, we have grown.

Probably the most gratifying thing, however, is the fact that most of life's minor crises don't faze us a bit. We save our sweat for the big ones, feeling fairly confident that the ways in which we've learned to cope will, once again, help us to transcend.

STEPS YOU CAN TAKE WITH YOUR FAMILY

- Identify role changes that have occurred in your family and discuss them with the family members involved.

- Read, study, and reach out for support as steps toward making the changes that will improve communication in your family relationships.

- Talk with others who are living with your chronic condition to learn how they cope. Share your own ideas.

- Talk with your family and friends about your feelings, and together brainstorm how you can reprioritize so that you have realistic goals for family life.

- Dare to address the sensitive areas of affection, intimacy and sexuality. First, sort through your own feelings, identify your needs, write them down, practice stating them, and then communicate them assertively.

- Recognize and capitalize on spontaneous moments.

- Develop your sense of humor.

- Live one day at a time.

7

MAINTAINING SELF-ESTEEM

When your body is not intact, it is especially important that your self-image remain whole and healthy. With physical impairment you are apt to be emotionally vulnerable, so this is the time to work hardest at keeping your self-esteem high. People may treat you as if you are invisible, or in a manner that infantalizes or smothers you. Also, you may be jeopardizing your own self-esteem in the ways you think and behave. It is interesting to learn how the survivors of illness and injury perceive themselves, how they handle it when they are confronted by assaults on their egos, and how they manage to build or preserve positive self concepts.

No easy answers or formulae exist. Everyone has to develop his or her own communication style for dealing with psychological affronts. However, the importance of dealing with them cannot be over-estimated. Whether you are able-bodied or physically challenged, if you yourself believe affronts and insults and take them to heart, they can erode your self-image and lower your self-esteem.

Self-perceptions

The first step in separating your illness from yourself is to recognize that you are not your disease. It can be helpful to use affirmations to this effect. For example, **I am not my arthritis. I am more than my illness. I am not my body. I am more than my body.**

Joseph Heller described how he perceived himself and his illness, Guillian-Barre, in *No Laughing Matter*:[1]

I never once throughout the entire experience thought of myself as weak, which to my mind means sleepy, lethargic, not strong. I was paralyzed, not weak. And in truth, I wasn't weak. My muscles were weak, I felt just fine during the day, with as much mental energy and zest as ever. It was the rest of me that was lousy and lying down on the job.

Two profiles are included in this chapter. Marguerite Webster, a blind counselor, and Cliff, a scientist, are also examples of the significance of self-perceptions in gaining transcendence over pain.

The Need to Take Assertive Action

Assertiveness training was first described in *Your Perfect Right: a Guide to Assertive Living*,[2] by Robert E. Alberti, and Michael L. Emmons. Their definition is:

Assertive behavior promotes equality in human relationships, enabling us to act in our own best interests, to stand up for ourselves without undue anxiety, to express honest feelings comfortably, to exercise personal rights without denying the rights of others.

The barriers to self-assertion are the belief that you don't have the **right** to be assertive, **anxiety** or **fearfulness** about being assertive, and a lack of **skills** for effective self-expression.

"Illness demands an active response," writes Cheri Register, in *Living With Chronic Illness: Days of Patience and Passion.*[3] "It does not deprive you of free will, even though it may very well limit your range of choices." When deciding how to preserve self-esteem, choices exist on the spectrum of giving up your autonomy at the one end, or stepping on other people to get what you want at the other. Awareness of the options in between can help you to feel less trapped. For example, to be passive is to allow yourself to become infantilized or invisible. It is giving up, taking to your bed, zonking yourself out on pills, and saying to your doctor, "Fix me." The other extreme is to refuse to give up anything--cigarettes, alcohol--and to refuse to follow medical recommendations. The assertive middle ground is to take responsibility for yourself with good self care skills--never giving up your control over whatever part of your life you can still manage, even if all that remains within your control is your emotional response to what is happening to you.

Rose, who suffers from chronic back pain, is an example of this. Her mother used to say, "Here, baby, let me help you get dressed. It hurts me to see you in so much pain." Rose would sigh, lie back, and let her mother minister to her. She chose to be passive. At other times she would assume an aggressive stance and scream at her mother. "When are you ever going to let me grow up! Why can't you ever leave me alone! Get out!" However, after her support group had a few sessions on assertiveness training, Rose managed to respond to her mother with a recognition of her good intentions, but a firm refusal. "Thank you, I'll call you when I need you," or "I appreciate your concern, but I really prefer to struggle with this chore myself," and "Mother, please don't call me 'baby' again. I'd like it if you would call me 'Rose.'" Rose now feels better. She realizes that with too much passivity she invariably becomes depressed, and that acting aggressively makes her feel guilty. When she manages to behave assertively, however, she feels better about herself and the relationship with her mother improves vastly. Assertiveness training can never guarantee the kind of response that you will get, but it does guarantee that you will feel better and stronger.

It's important to realize that caretakers and friends, such as Rose's mother, aren't being mean or intentionally trying to smother or elicit over-dependence. Their over-solicitousness and babying calls for just enough assertion to avoid the kind of traps that lead you to depression or guilt feelings. The same kind of response is called for when you are made to feel invisible--not passive resignation, not unbridled anger, but rather, an assertive, "Hey, I'm here. Let's interact, O.K.?" If the salesperson is directing his answers to the person who is pushing your wheel-chair instead of to you, rather than raging or giving up in despair, an "I beg your pardon, but I am the one who is making the purchase" will usually do.

Creating Your Environment

Another step on the path to enhanced self-esteem is to create an environment that is "user friendly." For example,

Amye Leong, who was mentioned earlier, the founder of a network of support groups for young people with arthritis,[4] and a sufferer of severe rheumatoid arthritis herself, has chosen office equipment (a computer, a conference telephone system, and other amenities) to help her function efficiently. If you're not familiar with computers, your doctor or occupational therapist can suggest many other technological devices to facilitate your daily tasks. You can also surround yourself with mementos or reminders of cheering thoughts that raise your spirits when you need it--anything from posters of rock singers to Biblical quotations, Hollywood nostalgia to family photographs, or landscapes to football pennants.

The friends and associates you choose to see are important, too. Allen Dyer in his book, *Your Erroneous Zones,* suggests that you note which of your friends and acquaintances are "toxic" to you and which are "nurturing." For example, Rose used to complain constantly about how inconsiderate and insensitive her sister was to her. When a friend asked why they spent so much time together, Rose suddenly realized that she hadn't considered limiting the amount of time she spent with her sister.

Perhaps you are not in a position to exert much control over your external environment. When that is your situation, taking charge of your inner environment is the challenge, albeit a difficult one. Whether you use prayer, the oldest form of meditation, or some form of bio-feedback, you can have an impact on your inner world, as many ex-prisoners of war and ex-hostages have discovered. Of course, this does not mean that you can by-pass grieving or pain, but it does mean that the pain is not compounded by feelings of total loss of control or loss of personal dignity. Thus, it may help, when you are evaluating your environment, to consider it on three levels--your physical surroundings, your friends, and your inner thoughts. Then you can assess how you can structure each of the three elements to enhance, rather than to inhibit, your life.

The Challenge to Educate

When people are awkward, tactless, or even cruel out of ignorance, it is a challenge to educate them. The education of others is another step you can take to raise your self-esteem. The hardest part about some diseases, such as lupus, chronic fatigue syndrome, and fibromyalgia, is that people don't understand or accept how ill you are because you look so well. To be constantly told that you look wonderful when you feel terrible can be trying. One such sufferer said that she can pick up the speaker's intent by the non-verbal clues. Sometimes the unspoken message is, "I don't understand how you can be so ill when you have such a healthy look. Please explain it to me." And so she does. Other times, however, the person is really saying, "I don't believe you. Why should I give you special treatment when you can't be that sick?" or, "You're using your illness. I think you're being lazy." When you are sure of what the feeling is behind the content of what is being said, then you can respond to that feeling. If it's lack of knowledge, you may provide information.

Responding to Insults, Slights and Affronts:

Suzette Haden Elgin, in *The Gentle Art of Verbal Self-Defense*,[5] outlines four basic skills needed for responding to insults:

1. Know when you are under attack.

2. Know what kind of attack you are facing.

3. Know how to make your defense fit the attack.

4. Know how to follow through.

For example, Rose's problem was that when her brother Bob called her a weakling, she did not see herself as being attacked. She just accepted that as a physically impaired person she was weak. Nor did she know that she was facing a bullying attack. If she had, Rose might have retorted that in her case it was only her muscles that were weak. She might even have suggested that they play a game like Scrabble in order to underscore her strength. When she learns how to rise above insults, Rose will no longer allow herself to be victimized.

Another example is Susan. Severe back and knee problems made it imperative that Susan lose weight. Her counselor suggested that she ask her husband to give her positive reinforcement for her efforts. She returned the following week and said, "Tom's involved. He told me he could see that I was losing weight because my arms look all withered." Susan didn't even realize that she had been attacked. With further help from her therapist, she was able to confront him with, "Isn't there some other aspect of my weight loss that you can choose to respond to?"

Again, Rose is an example. When her mother told the doctor that her daughter was too immature to handle her medication, Rose, if she were operating passively, would buy into this demeaning view of her capacity to manage. Or, if she were to become aggressive, she could shout, "I may be immature, but I'm not as stupid (or as insensitive, or as bossy), as you are!" But that is hardly recommended for improving the quality of relationships. An assertive response might be, "I'm ready to take it on now. Thanks, anyway."

Sometimes, however, group action is needed to encourage public education and community action. As described in Chapter 10, Sonda Aronson started an organization to educate the public about disabled artists, Neil Marcus developed a newsletter, and the Danets initiated a movement called Partnerships for A Better Community.

These strategies can be used in a wide variety of situations, and it takes judgment to know which strategy to apply in response to which challenge. The following chart may guide you in making some of those determinations.

STRATEGIES FOR MAINTAINING YOUR SELF-ESTEEM

CHALLENGE	STRATEGY
To improve self-perceptions	USE AFFIRMATIONS and your inner dialogue to see yourself as more than your illness.
To counter infantilization	AFFIRM YOUR ADULTHOOD assertively (not passively or aggressively).
To respond when you're being made to feel invisible	TAKE ASSERTIVE ACTION to make yourself seen and heard.
To create your own environment	MAKE AN ASSESSMENT of your needs on all three levels. Devise a plan to meet as many as you can.

To answer ignorant/tactless questions	**BECOME CHALLENGED TO TEACH**; practice different educational approaches until you find one that works for you.
To confront deliberate discrimination	**JOIN A LOBBYING GROUP**, learn your rights, write your legislators, take social action.

It takes skills to develop a style of communication that protects and nourishes your self-esteem, skills that can be learned with practice and determination as illustrated in the following profiles of Marguerite and Cliff. Both work on their self-perceptions and create their own environments taking advantage of what has been called "uninvited opportunity." Refusing to be victims despite severe physical impairments, they experiment with educational approaches, and they assert their rights effectively. They are also good examples of countering depression, coping with pain, and many other attributes that lead out of victimization and into a restoration of a sense of self. High self-esteem is the underpinning upon which many of the other attributes are built, no matter what is happening to your body. Keeping your self-esteem high is a giant step toward transcendence.

Marguerite: Woman of Vision

Marguerite, 41, is a family therapist with a thriving private practice and infectious enthusiasm about her work. She dresses beautifully, has lovely skin, and is so composed and deft that it's hard to believe that she's blind.

Her vision problem started when she was a junior in high school and began to experience the deterioration of night vision. After endless visits to specialists she was diagnosed with retinitis pigmentosa, a diagnosis that was so new that she had to spell it out for some ophthalmologists.

Marguerite lost most of her sight when she was sixteen years old, going from 20/20 vision to 20/200 (which constitutes legal blindness). Her desire to be like her peers was so intense that to be different was to be devastated, so she went to phenomenal extremes to cover up her visual impairment. When she went down steps that she could barely see, she would fumble in her purse so that if she did trip, people would think that it was because she was distracted. When she could no longer recognize faces, she pretended to be reading a book so her friends wouldn't think that she was snubbing them. She could have used large print books, but, she says, "You can't be forty-one at sixteen, and at that time, everything was focused on how I could seem sighted."

On dates, in dark restaurants or bars, she couldn't see well enough to get to the Ladies' Room without stumbling against tables or staggering a bit. She would appear to be slightly drunk, or stoned, which in that age group in the sixties, was much more acceptable than being physically impaired.

In her senior year, when faced with having to take the New York State Regents' exams, under time pressure, a teacher read the questions to her to save time. Marguerite told her friends she'd just taken it in another room. "And I would not use a cane. Go on a date and use a cane? Forget it!" she says.

Few resources were available in those days, "Not that I would have used them anyway," she adds, ruefully. Because Marguerite and her father were both in denial, her mother had to be discreet in finding out what was available. Her dad still has a difficult time accepting that she's blind. He says, "She's fine, look at her, she's doing great."

"Things happen for different reasons," Marguerite believes. "Career choices were so limited for the visually impaired, and I didn't come from a wealthy family, so my mother engineered it so I could go to college and major in speech therapy. I worked in that field for three years, and then with financial help from State Rehabilitation went to graduate school. My first Master's Degree was in Special Education, working with the visually impaired. I love school. I would have been a secretary and had a different life, but education opened doors for me."

Marguerite now has three specializations: work with the speech impaired, the visually impaired, and the developmentally disabled, but she doesn't want to be stereotyped as doing only that kind of work. She also knows that the underlying problems of people who are in pain are pretty much the same.

Being a blind therapist, however, involves heavy expenses. Marguerite has a reader, a secretary, and a driver, but she views them as she would rent--necessary overhead expenses. Because she has developed a good reputation and referral base, she can cover those expenses.

Although Marguerite is a skillful therapist who deals with a variety of clients with a wide range of problems, she does have superior knowledge and expertise in working with both partially sighted and blind clients. She says that, in general, people can understand blindness much better than they can being partially sighted. The partially sighted are a group that has been neglected, she feels, and are in "a completely different ball-park with a whole different set of adjustments to make."

Marguerite has been totally blind for the last six years, yet she appears very comfortable within herself. She says that dependence can be seen as a weakness within ourselves, but "when I am clear and at peace, those perceptions don't bother me--I don't have to be a 'little guru' about blindness. I will sit with you and be really with you--give you honesty about myself--but I don't have to have all the answers."

Ed, Marguerite's husband of 18 years, has made many career changes, too, going from teaching to engineering to politics to writing. She says, "I would change anything in my life in order to be able to see again--anything--except my marriage. I would not change that." She and Ed have often wondered about their "luck" at having such a strong marriage and have concluded that it is due to how supportive they are of each other, especially through all the changes in their lives.

Marguerite says that she was able to let go of her need to pretend when it became too exhausting. One turning point occurred while she was lecturing to a junior high school class and a 13 year old girl asked her, "If God decided that he would let you be able to see again, would you want to? Not that you need to--you're doing just fine." That's when it hit her that she was leaving out all of the anger and frustration, that she wasn't giving people the total picture. She answered that <u>of course</u> she would want to see again.

"At that point I became able to give up my need to be the super-educator and super-role model. I could be more honest, and I could be myself." She developed a more authentic self-perception and the skills to maintain her self-esteem. That's one reason she comes across not only as charming and helpful, but also as quite comfortable with her restored self.

Self esteem is built throughout a lifetime. It is built by parents and other significant people such as teachers who encourage us, giving loving support. It is developed through having success in learning and applying skills that bring personal satisfaction. Both Marguerite and Cliff, whose story follows, seem to have entered adolescence with high enough self-esteem to see them through those teen years when self identity was shifting, and new diagnoses were being made.

Each person enters crisis with differing degrees of self-esteem. Whatever yours is at this time, to learn how others cope can be interesting, and might help you to enhance your own self-esteem.

Cliff: Computer as Metaphor for Mind

Cliff has lived 44 years with ankylosing spondylitis, an inflammatory disease of the spine. Over many years the spine develops deposits of calcium along it's ligaments ultimately resulting in a stiff board-like or bamboo spine. His illness first appeared when he was 13 years old and his joints started swelling, making it difficult for him to walk. He was misdiagnosed as having rheumatic fever and stayed in bed for six months.

"This was quite an education," he says. "All of a sudden you're out of it. You go for months without seeing your friends. But it's the only ball game in town, so you learn to play it." He'd known some physically disabled people whose "personalities were disasters, and in no way did I want to turn out like them. At that age you are flexible, and I developed technical interests." Science always interested him, and reading was one of his mainstays. In addition, he was elected president of his high school class, was voted outstanding student, and was also the salutatorian.

These achievements built his self-esteem, which carried over into adulthood, and subsequent successes further contributed to his independence and to his positive self-perceptions. He has rarely let depression get the best of him in spite of the two major tragedies in his life, the onset of his illness, and his brother's death in World War II, which happened at about the same time in his life.

High Risk Surgery

Now, at 57, Cliff looks like Santa Claus would look if Santa were thinner, had red hair, and a bushy red beard. There is jolliness about him, and his smile is almost a chortle. He talks matter-of-factly about all that he's been through, such as the episode he experienced ten years ago. He was forced to quit work because he was on so much medication that his stomach just couldn't handle it; anything that seemed to help the arthritis was disastrous to his stomach. In addition,his body was so bent over he spent most of the time in a wheel-chair. He couldn't tell who was in a room unless he was sitting down because he couldn't raise his head to look around. His spine had completely calcified except for one joint in his neck between the first and second cervical vertebra, the Axis and the Atlas. The body's post-like structure, which attaches the tendons which control head motion, had disintegrated. The result was that his head drooped to his chest, limiting how far he could open his mouth, and painfully pinching nerves to his scalp and the back of his neck causing pain. At his home computer he had to "peek over the edge of the keyboard." Finally it became difficult even to open his mouth.

The doctors were waiting until he couldn't take the pain any more because the surgery was so risky; there was a ten percent chance that he would not make it through the surgery, and a ten per cent chance of ending up on a respirator. He did survive the surgeries, which consisted of a neck fusion with halo traction and the breaking and fusion of the middle and lower spine, using Harrington rods for support. (These rods are stainless steel, an eighth of an inch in diameter, about fourteen inches long, and are attached to his spine. They have little hook-like appendages that attach to the vertebrae and cannot be removed until the back is healed.) It meant two years in a body jacket made of plastic and strapped on with velcro--warm and uncomfortable. But to Cliff, "Coming out straight was like being born again."

Relationship with Doctor

Cliff has a "long-term doctor for a long-term illness," an internist specializing in rheumatology who also teaches at the University of Southern California. He referred Cliff to the U.S.C. Los Angeles County Rancho Los Amigos Medical Center, which specializes in rheumatic diseases, spinal injury and deformity disciplines. There Cliff attends a rheumatology clinic regularly, where the medication is prescribed for the next few months. They referred him to the arthritis surgical group for his neck fusion, who, in turn referred him to the spinal deformity group for his spinal osteotomies.

Medication

Cliff is well aware of the medical trade-offs of the different arthritis medications, some of which have strong side effects. "Some pain medications have less side effects but don't help the disease. It becomes a compromise for an acceptable quality of life with acceptable risk. Each time the arthritis worsens, I experiment until I'm convinced I have a good combination. At one time, I was using nine different medications; I'm now using five with higher discomfort but less risk."

Computer Analogy to the Brain

But perhaps Cliff's chief coping mechanism is his unique view of the brain. He is thoughtful and logical, and consciously uses his mind to deal with his physical pain. "The brain," explains Cliff, "is like a large number of computers working simultaneously, comparing the sensory data coming from the eyes, ears, and other senses with the way the brain perceives the world. This is all done subconsciously using learned programs. We don't have to think about it. However, feelings are signals from the subconscious to the conscious that the comparison between what is expected and what exists does not match. The conscious then takes over and tries to identify what caused the feeling and take corrective action, either by changing the world or by changing the brain's perception of the world. Feelings must operate very rapidly (fear reflex action) and independently of language." You can thus have some control over chronic pain, according to Cliff's theory, in that you can cover it up by thinking or doing something else.

"Of course," he acknowledges, "there are times when the pain is so strong that it blocks everything else out. During those periods there is no way that you can possibly do anything else." But Cliff believes that most of the time you can exert quite a bit of mental control over pain.

"I find when I go sailing I have very little pain. It's a matter of how your brain is interpreting what is going on and of doing what you want to do instead of giving in to it." **Peace and Quiet** is the name of his sailboat. He says that out on the water the pain almost goes away.

Cliff conceptualizes depression as getting into a program that you can't get out of, a "closed loop" in computer language. He explains that if behaviors are learned, they cannot be forgotten. You can only lay another program on top of the former one so that you don't use the one that's there. That's why he doesn't think it's productive to dwell on what caused things in the past or that you can free yourself from anger by talking about it. He thinks it's more helpful to learn something new.

As for anger, Cliff says "It's useful to tell me what I don't know." To him it's an indicator, or a clue, that he needs to learn more about handling a situation.

Independence

These well thought-out views of life give Cliff a sense of control and independence. He speaks sadly of the patients at the rehabilitation hospital, some in their twenties, who acted as if they were two years old emotionally. Their parents filled all their needs, including many that they could have met on their own. When they were hospitalized, they tried to get their nurses to baby them, too.

Cliff is so independent that he does not believe there is value in staying close to others when you are in a lot of pain--not family, not close friends and least of all, support groups. To him the supposed value in that kind of mutual support is a myth. "It's a matter of backing off when it's necessary. As long as I'm around people who feel sorry for me, I don't get anything done." At 22, after completing two years of college, he left his home in Minnesota and moved to California to become more independent. He deliberately rented a third-floor apartment so he would be forced to walk up the stairs even though it was painful. "If you're going to hurt," says Cliff, "You might as well be where you want to be."

Career and Family

Cliff spent most of his career at the California Institute of Technology Jet Propulsion Laboratory, beginning as an electronic technician. He left, after 23 years, as a senior engineer. His first project was supervising the fabrication of the transmitters which were to fly on the first U.S. satellites. Later he worked on advanced electronic research projects including lasers, masers, atomic frequency standards, microwave equipment (patent), and evaluated new discoveries in electronics for use in deep space communications.

Cliff married Virginia in 1970. They adopted a boy and a girl, now 20 and 22, and he says they could not possibly have had two finer children than the two they were privileged to raise.

Cliff transcends because he believes there needs to be a separation of mental functions from the physical body. He sees the body as the platform of the mind. If your existence is based on using your mind, then, if everything else deteriorates, you still have your mind. Then problems with your body are not going to take you down.

Cliff is not one to be taken down. He believes that if you can't work, you can always learn or "lay on another program." Cliff's self-esteem remains high because he uses his mind and his multiple skills to transcend the pain of his physical body.

The stories of Marguerite and Cliff demonstrate that people cope quite differently. Their perceptions of what is acceptable may vary; they tell themselves different things. What they have in common, and what people have in common who are restoring their sense of themselves, is that their adjustment and growth comes from positive self-talk. Their focus is on building on their strengths.

STEPS YOU CAN TAKE TO RAISE YOUR SELF-ESTEEM

- List ten qualities that you like in yourself and write them in the form of affirmations. (Examples: I have a good sense of humor and will continue to use it. I have a good imagination and apply it to imaging. I write well and enjoy recording my successes).

- Put this list in a handy place and read it regularly.

- Identify relationships or situations where you would like to be more assertive. Plan a relevant assertive (not aggressive) request, write it down, and practice asking it out loud.

- Evaluate your environment--your physical surroundings, friends, and inner thoughts. Then assess how you might restructure each of these three elements to enhance your life.

NOTES

8

CULTIVATING REFLECTIVE SKILLS

When mobility is curtailed and frustrations accumulate with a terrifying momentum, one of the greatest fears is of loss of control of your body, your activities, your life. Reflective skills are tools for recapturing a sense of control, and although at first developing these tools appears to be a hard job, it is relatively easy. And they really work as steps toward restoring that sense of control.

Jung used the concept of "doing inner work" to describe looking inside yourself for insight and peace of mind. The reflective skills discussed in this chapter: imagery, keeping a journal, and life review accomplish this. Although briefly described here, reflective skills also include dreamwork and meditation. It is often useful to join a group or find a teacher when beginning to use these skills, since there are steps to follow to obtain maximum benefit.

Imagery

Pain clinics suggest that you use fantasy to gain control over your pain. You will recall from the chapter on pain that Marsha could separate herself from it by visualizing herself floating on a cloud away from her body. Cliff visualized his brain as a computer that he could program. Some people give their pain a color, or a personality in the form of an animal or bird that they can communicate with and tell to go away. Others can imagine their pain into some form that they can get rid of by burning it up or dumping it in the ocean.

Carolyn Engel who lives with three concommitant diseases, systemic lupus, cerebrospinal fluid rhinorrhea, and a heart problem, describes the process for her as learning to quiet her mind so that she can connect with the power of her mind to help make her body healthier. In a group activity she drew a picture of her pain at its worst, and then again demonstrating how she would change the image to show how the pain would look if it were tolerable. In the first instance there are arrows piercing her body and a two thousand pound weight on her head. In the second picture the weight is reduced to twenty pounds, a smile has replaced a frown, and there are a fraction as many arrows. The heart is giving out positive vibrations instead of being pierced with pain. After going through exercises in relaxation and guided imagery in which she created healing and restorative pictures, she responded to a question about what she had learned about herself:

> Drawing my pain helped me get to know it better. It helped me be less afraid of the pain and gave me the courage to go into it and to work through it.
>
> I have more control over my pain than I realized.

Journaling

Recording how you feel is an excellent method of developing reflective your skills. Your journal may or may not include illustrations or drawings. An anecdotal diary that is an accumulation of factual accounts of day-to-day happenings is not recommended. That kind of record does not yield insights or lead to self-understanding. Instead, keep a dream log, a running description of your emotional responses to your illness, or a record of your progress in imaging. Helen Keller, in her journal, *Midstream; My Later Life*,[1] says, "One's life story cannot be told with complete veracity. A true autobiography would have to be written in states of mind, emotions, heartbeats, smiles and tears, not in months and years, or physical events. Life is marked off on the soul-chart by feelings, not by dates." So don't let your editing, censoring left brain restrict the flow. Your journal does not have to be historical to be useful. Some diarists write solely to clarify their thoughts. "How do I know what I think, until I see what I say?" says W. H. Auden.

Your journal accomplishes many purposes. Probably the most important one is that when it is properly focused, it will raise your self-esteem. To get started, think about a time in your life when you felt a sense of achievement--when you accomplished something that made you feel elated, powerful, wanting to celebrate. It can be a simple thing, like when your kindergarten teacher looked at the picture you crayoned and said, "That's a nice house." It can be when you earned your Ph.D., or caught your first fish, when you had your first baby or got your driver's license. The point is to relive and enjoy the feelings and the realization that you can feel those feelings again, that you are the same person who experienced that joy. Getting in touch with your feelings is the first step in journaling.

Eric Berne, who wrote *Games People Play*, suggests a "Gold Stamp Theory." You can collect memories to savor when you are down, or you can feed your depression by collecting what he calls "dirty brown stamps," the disappointments, failures, insults and bummers. A certain number of dirty brown stamps entitles you to a divorce; a million or so to a suicide attempt. The only point to the theory is that you can ask yourself whether you want to be a dirty brown stamp collector or a gold stamp collector. Your journal is your gold stamp collection to bring out and savor when you need it.

Keeping your journal helps your self-esteem in other ways, too. Dr. James E. Burrin of the University of Southern California explains, "There is a personal adjustment between the ideal self and the actual self." In the course of writing about one's life, "The actual self goes up in one's estimation and the ideal self is lowered somewhat so that it is more realistic and attainable. The result is that the person is more at peace; there's less tension and anxiety." All the "what-might-have-beens" become reconciled with the "what is."

To get that balanced self-concept your journal certainly cannot be all sweetness and light. It is a place to vent pent-up feelings, negative as well as positive, thus lowering your stress level.

> *Give sorrow words, the grief*
> *That does not speak*
> *Knits up the o'erwrought breast*
> *And bids it break.*

> *MacBeth*

We all yearn to be the agents of change instead of the victims of it, and when illness victimizes, the rage has to have an outlet or it tears at our bodies along with the disease.

As an outlet, your journal is a place of safety. In speech and other behavior you run the risk of being destructive to yourself or others, deliberately or inadvertently. But you can write letters, and then tear them up--or not. You can confide in your diary where the only risk is a prying eye. When deprived of physical outlets like batting a ball, running, or long hikes in the out-of-doors, writing is available, and serves the purpose if you can find your own free-flowing style. You can choose to keep it private or to share it.

Life Review as a Part of Your Journal

"Life Review" is a concept that was developed by the eminent geriatric psychiatrist, Robert Butler.[1] He theorizes that reminiscing serves a purpose; it is not just idle rumination characteristic of the aging and portending senility, but rather an adaptive function providing psychological preparation for the next phase of one's life. In studies, the fact that there is a tendency for non-depressed subjects to reminisce more than depressed subjects would seem to substantiate that it does serve such a purpose. He cites many examples of members of Life Review Groups who used autobiographical writing as a step in the resolution of grief and toward giving meaning to their lives. He recommends that such groups include adults of all ages and gives poignant examples of the bridging of generation gaps through the use of this approach.

The purpose is to make reminiscence more conscious, deliberate, efficient, and often, enjoyable. The tools you use can be scrap books, albums, old letters, pilgrimages, reunions; anything that puts you in touch with your past. There are no rules, but it is important that you concentrate on what is important to you, not on what you think should be important according to somebody else's criteria, and that you emphasize feelings rather than facts. Writing skills, or the lack of them, are not important.

Journal Therapy

Ira Progoff developed a similar approach which he calls "Journal Therapy". He describes it in *At A Journal Workshop*[2] as an ongoing, open-ended program of personal growth. "The effective principle operating in this (the intensive journal) is that, when a person is shown how to reconnect himself with the contents and the continuity of his life, the inner thread of movement by which his life has been unfolding reveals itself to him by itself. Given the opportunity, a life crystallizes out of its own nature, revealing its meaning and its goal." One section in the process of his Intensive Journal involves a "Life History Log; Stepping Stones; Intersections; Roads Taken and Not Taken."

Focusing on turning points is also recommended by the Swiss psychiatrist, Paul Tournier in his book, *Learn To Grow Old.*[3] According to him the richness in experience lies in those decisive moments when your life is turned in a new direction. In every life there are a few special moments that count for more than all the rest because they meant the taking of a stand, a self-commitment, a decisive choice. "It is commitment that creates the person. It is by commitment that man reveals his humanity. The turning points of life are generally few in number. They may have been slow, almost unconscious, gradually brought to fruition through extended crises, or they may have been like the flash of lightning, the sudden burst into consciousness of a process worked through in the subconscious. Yet, when we try to understand their essential character we perceive that they are always an encounter: encounter with an idea or encounter with a person, before which the subject cannot remain neutral. He simply had to take sides, to shoulder responsibility, to commit himself.... Encounter with a man, a friend, a book, a film, a fact of nature, a philosopher, a teacher--suddenly the whole gamble of life is embodied in a particular encounter which confers on life its whole meaning and all its creative power."

When beginning your journal, therefore, you may want to think about the major turning points in your life and if they indeed did come as a result of an encounter. The concept of turning points is expanded upon in Chapter 12, **Identifying Turning Points**. Perhaps one of your encounters was your encounter with your illness, or with the doctor who made the diagnosis, or with a role model who transcended the suffering from that illness.

Some people prefer to start by thinking of their life as a branching tree. What are your roots, and what are the major branching points in the development of your life? And then there are those who prefer to choose a theme. Do you want to record your dreams, the history of your health/body, your emotional ups and downs, or the story of your career?

Writing autobiographically, or "Life Review" leads to your finding purpose and meaning in your life. Victor Frankl wrote, "A human being cannot live a life without meaning; if the meaning is trivial, the life will be trivial; if the meaning is exalted, the life will be exalted--one is free to choose. Not to choose results in an 'existential vacuum' that is life destroying." A Journal won't guarantee exaltation, but it will go a long way toward filling that "existential vacuum" and making you feel better about your life and your situation.

Janice Harris Lord in *No Time For Good-byes*,[4] emphasized that writing can be therapeutic, "Writing can uncover lost or repressed feelings which need expression.... Another valuable aspect of writing is that it provides a tool for measuring progress. It helps to look at what one wrote three months ago or six months ago and compare it with the present."

Again, your journal can serve many purposes, but is especially beneficial for raising self-esteem, releasing pent-up feelings, and for life review. If you keep a journal it won't be long before you will feel it working as a step toward restoring a sense of control over your life. It is your log of your journey in inner space and helps you survive, cope, and even transcend the pain of chronic illness.

The following profile of Elsa illustrates the use of several reflective skills. Through meditating and keeping a journal she gives voice to her intuition and gains a sense of control over her life.

Elsa: Blind Terror

Elsa Campbell[5] is a self-assured, vibrant young woman with shiny dark hair, a pleasant, hearty voice and an infectious laugh. She has insulin dependent diabetes. Among the many complications of that disease, blindness was always her greatest fear. A low point came at age 31 when she developed proliferative diabetic retinopathy. She experienced a series of retinal hemorrhages. Each time the retina bled she had to look through pools of, "black, spotted, murky junk," realizing that the disease process might go on until there was no vision left.

Elsa was diagnosed as diabetic when she was eleven years old. Issues of control are especially poignant with childhood diabetics. Elsa wrote: "Regardless of the threats of blindness and destruction to the organs of my body I still could not master the strict regimen that was required to be in 'good control.'" It is now admitted by diabetologists that it is nearly impossible to keep a normal blood sugar using the diabetes regimen prescribed in the 1960s and 70s.

Elsa explains,"An ideal was asserted that I could not live up to. This was the first of many betrayals by the medical profession that I have experienced. Their knowledge was partial, but it was turned into an ideal formula that in their model of the human body should have worked. I was lectured many times that one injection of insulin along with the proper diet would be the key to good control. What came across to me was that all good disciplined diabetics should be able to accomplish this nebulous concept of good control. Even today it is not known how high blood sugar has to be before damage begins to occur in the body. For some people it is much lower than others. I naturally thought there must be something terribly wrong with my character since I usually failed to have negative urine tests, that is, no sugar spilling out of the kidneys. Constant failure at not being able to do it right just led to apathy and self-loathing for not being perfect. The problem of not reaching perfection weighs on your mind even more as you realize your imperfection leads to blindness and deteriorating health...

"When my ophthalmologist told me I had retinopathy I had to deal with my feelings along with coming to terms with the diagnosis. I do not wonder that the research literature states that many diabetics deny the diagnosis of retinopathy, and therefore do not get proper care. Much more than just the vision loss must be dealt with. Denial protects the ego against unwanted or over-whelming emotion. The denial can exist in family members and the medical profession as well as the patient."

Intuition and Meditation

A time comes when you no longer deny, but begin to cope. With Elsa, this came when she listened to her intuition, and used meditation and other reflective skills to find answers to problems of control over her blood sugar. She cautions diabetics that

126

meditation lowers blood sugar and should be used with awareness.

It is natural for Elsa to look inward. She grew up in a family where the unspoken rules were: "Don't feel, don't trust, and don't share." She learned to turn to her own inner self for direction. By the time she was a teenager she had learned that she could pop a question into her mind and using her own natural intuition, eventually an answer would come to her. Now, as an adult, she says, " I define a problem, think about it, let go, and wait patiently for answers. They come in different ways. I might have a hunch to talk with a particular person, read a book, or attend a lecture. An answer might come to me while doing the dishes, or in a dream." By trusting her intuition and meditating upon a problem, Elsa gains control and finds ways to deal with the emotional impact of dealing with diabetic complications.

During a time in her early thirties when control was elusive, a pastor at Elsa's church said, "Write. Keep a notebook. It will help you deal with your feelings." Elsa said, "When I saw my thoughts and feelings on paper, instead of being in a huge crisis, I saw that problems were being resolved. The events of my life began to fit together. I could see how I'd coped. My past was right there on paper and it helped me cope in the present. I realized my life was moving in a positive direction. I sensed God, or a higher power working in my life."

The state-of-the-art technology of the 1980s is helping Elsa monitor her own blood sugar levels, and to administer insulin accordingly. This is a giant step in gaining a feeling of control over her body and her life. She combines practical goal-oriented learning and reflective skills to help her cope with stress, fear, helplessness and anger. She is an insightful and independent thinker. One of the many creative ways that she coped with her anxiety was to devote her master's thesis to how she came to terms with her fear of blindness. She has generously lent her report, "Healing the Trauma of Diabetic Vision Loss," for this profile.

Over the years Elsa has sought help from a diabetic psychiatrist, has worked both as a volunteer and a staff member of a hospice to find out how people handle death, and has volunteered her considerable skills with the American Diabetes Association. She is married and is raising a daughter. Her present goals are to develop local resources for the blind, and to finish her internship as a Marriage, Family & Child Counselor. A more long term goal is to write a book, and when she does it will reach deep into the hearts of the large numbers of people who face blindness.

STEPS YOU CAN TAKE TO DEEPEN YOUR REFLECTIVE SKILLS

- Reflect on what you have just read. Experiment with different techniques, or choose a method that is right for you now. Different methods may work for you at different times.

- Create a comforting imagery. Visualize a serene scene--your favorite place to relax, a comforting scene from your childhood, or a place of great natural beauty and peace. Escape into it and enjoy it.

- Get a notebook and some pens and pencils.

- Reminisce about an incident when you experienced a sense of achievement. Write down how you felt, whether you wanted to laugh, or cry, or hug someone. Write a few sentences recalling the experience. **You have started your journal!**

- Collect memories of awards, achievements, complements, and record them in your journal.

- Set aside time each day to develop your reflective skills. To begin with, ten to twenty minutes is enough time to begin to form the habit.

- Join a journal, meditation, or dreamwork group for further support and skill building.

NOTES

9

REACHING OUT FOR SUPPORT

Everyone needs some kind of support system. Your family can be one. Your friends and fellow workers can be available to you. Another person with the same condition can be of help. At some point, you may find a support group is a place to gain information, coping skills, and emotional support. You may have questions: What should I look for in a support group? How do they work? What are the benefits? Are there drawbacks? This chapter addresses these questions.

Even the Surgeon General of the United States, C. Everett Koop, has acknowledged the need, and endorsed increased use of self-help groups. "Curing and repairing are no longer enough. They are only part of the total health care that most people require....I believe in self-help as an effective way of dealing with problems, stress, hardship and pain...." The self-help support group is one of America's fastest-growing methods of coping with personal problems.

The rapid rise of support groups in this country results from basic social changes that have caused alienation, or lack of opportunity for intimate relationships. Examples of these social changes are the modifications in the structure of the family, people's increased mobility, and urbanization.

A support group is one which you can count on for non-judgmental acceptance and encouragement, and that will keep your discussion in confidence. An infinite variety of support groups are available. They range from heterogeneous groups that are loosely structured to those that are limited to people with the same specific problems and that have preplanned highly structured formats. Many Anonymous groups exist--the first was Alcoholics Anonymous--that give support to people with specific needs. There are clubs and fraternal organizations that have nationwide support systems. Some families function as support groups and some church clubs, Bible study classes and other religious bodies serve the same purpose. There are groups for teens, parents, seniors, weight control, quitting-smoking, writing, job-seeking, marriage enrichment, and many others.

It's important to note that the terms "self-help group" and "support group" are often used interchangeably. Also, the distinction between a "therapy group" and a "self-help group" is unclear and the overlap is great. Their goals are information gathering, emotional support, modeling, goal setting, insight, growth, and self-esteem raising.

Support groups fulfill a need of people with chronic illnesses because of the isolation that illness can cause, and because of widespread misunderstandings about illness. There is also need for support groups for spouses and families of chronically ill people. Such groups are starting up all over the United States to meet this need. Combined meetings work well, especially when the program involves instruction about the disease. However, joint meetings should not take the place of meetings for you, the chronically ill. You need a place to ventilate and to share with people who "have been there."

The purpose of support groups is to provide emotional support for members in a safe environment, and to provide a forum for the discussion of feelings and the interchange of ideas and information that will help its members cope with their illness. Most ongoing support groups benefit from professional leadership because leaderless groups tend to peter out over time. A leader sets a tone to avoid the pitfalls of too much depressive talk, lack of direction, or uneven participation. Whoever runs your group should have skills as a facilitator and be well versed in the problems of your illness. Research on groups suggests eight as the ideal size but in actuality anything from three to fifty has been known to work well. The advantage of small groups is the heightened opportunity for participation. On the other hand, larger groups that are educationally oriented are apt to have greater access to experts in their field of interest.

Group counseling offers some advantages that are not found in one-to-one therapy. In groups there are more sources of feed-back, more points of view expressed, and more interchange. In addition, groups provide multiple models for various styles of communicating with family members, medical personnel, and others. Also group feed-back carries more impact and is often taken more seriously than feed-back from a counselor alone. However, groups are not a substitute for individual therapy and are best used as supplementary to it.

The advantages of combining people who have "been there" a long time with those whose onset is recent usually outweigh the advantages of separating recent-onset participants from "old-timers." The latter become role models and gain from being able to be helpful. Some groups come up with quite original approaches to championing their members. Some artists have a group that has a prayer breakfast before any one of its members exhibits his work. The "Professional Women's Pig-Out Group" in Sacramento met one Sunday a month to eat all day and talk about their problems.

Some groups are much more confrontive than others such as drug rehabilitation groups that are designed to challenge strong anti-social defenses. Some groups are more task-oriented, some more educationally focused, and some have emotional support as

133

their only goal. Self-help groups that are designed for persons with specific diseases usually have emotional support as their primary goal, which is appropriate.

Experience has shown that people with chronic illnesses have much to gain from participating in support groups. Those who have similar problems and are willing to share their experience can be incredibly supportive. However, this does not mean that a support group is for everyone, or that every support group is successful.

Some ill people who have transcended their pain feel that a support group is not appropriate for them. Others make excellent use of support groups for certain phases of their illnesses, and then go on to other kinds of interactions with people. Many who have been recently diagnosed believe that they are not ready for that kind of participation until they are further along in their journey. You may feel like the author of the following poem:

DENIAL

Don't tell me I should seek help.
I don't want to go;
I don't want to know.

It is all still so new -
If I go to a group
I'll be telling myself it's true;
> *And I have to listen to someone*
> *else's problems.*

I'd rather hide,
Thank you - - for now,
Behind my facade
And tell myself I'm getting better
- That the doctors might be wrong
- That the lab was mistaken

I'll bide my time
Until <u>*I'm*</u> *ready.*

> *Where else do I have control?*

Joyce Dace-Lombard

Sometimes seeing people in the later stages of an illness feeds fear of the future. For example there are multiple sclerosis groups that have divided themselves into two levels; earlier and recent onset as the problems of the two groups are seen as being quite different. In other situations, the more seasoned members learn to put the newcomers at ease and the newcomers appreciate being able to learn from the survivors' experiences.

If you are not ready to join a group, some self-help organizations provide one-to-one support from a person who has the same illness, someone who has survived and can understand what you are going through in a way that others cannot.

Benefits

Those who are benefiting from groups have reported the following gains:

- Acceptance of me as an O.K. person.
- Validation of my feelings; that I am not lazy, crazy, or neurotic, and that it's not, "all in my head."
- The feeling that I'm not alone, not isolated.
- Socialization and new friendships.
- Networking; learning about doctors, relevant articles, other groups and community resources.
- Perspective; feed-back about my expectations so that I can keep them realistic.
- Re-enforcement for efforts toward positive action.
- Encouragement that keeps me energized.
- Help with goal setting.
- Improved communication skills.
- Training to be more assertive with medical personnel, family members, employer, colleagues, and others.
- Help with grieving the losses.
- Help in countering depression.
- Help in dealing with pain.
- Help in becoming better informed about my disease.

In support groups which deal with disability, issues of age, educational level, and social status seem to melt away because of the overriding concerns of coping with the illness. Co-educational groups are usually recommended. However, under certain circumstances same-sex sub-groups are indicated because of the reluctance of some people to speak of bodily functions in the presence of the opposite sex. Also, sometimes women tend to clam up, compete for, or start nurturing the men in the group.

Some support groups have a curriculum for a set number of sessions. This eliminates time-wasting and trial and error. Another advantage is that everyone in the group starts at the same time, repetition is avoided and the older members don't have to hear the same stories repeated. On the other hand, an open-ended group (ongoing) means that openings are always available. You don't have to wait, sometimes several months, for the next group to begin. The overlapping provides opportunities for older members to orient new members by telling how the group has helped them. This re-enforces the gains that have been made, and as stated above, provides good modeling.

In planning the content of meetings, bear two things in mind. First, ensure that the members participate in the decisions about how the meetings are to be run and what topics are to be covered. This can be done by circulating questionnaires, having their suggestions recorded on a blackboard for discussion, or by a program committee. Compromises may be necessary. For example, one segment might want a task-oriented channel for political action and another faction might be pulling for meditation, both viable alternatives that warrant consideration. Secondly, there needs to be balance between structure and instruction on the one hand, and ventilation and open unrestricted sharing on the other.

You can learn from role models, and you can also be one. After living through your experience with your illness you are in a position to help others who are confronted with similar challenges. A woman living with diabetes wrote,[1]

> *As you talk with someone else with diabetes, you will find that not only your anger and frustration about diabetes will disappear, but you can take pride in the fact that you are doing well. In a sense your are a member of a unique community of individuals whose condition has given them a special knowledge about living that is helpful to everyone.... Once you realize this and put your knowledge to work you will acquire a sense of satisfaction in taking charge not only of your diabetes, but of life itself.*

It is important that you assess your need for support and make decisions about where to look for it. There are many options: you may choose to seek support from a friend, a religious counselor, therapist, an individual volunteer at the society or foundation set up to help people with your illness, or a support group.

Support groups can be effective in helping you move from victim through survival to transcending the pain of chronic illness. If one isn't available, consider starting one. The resources listed in the appendix can provide further information about what groups are available in your area, and how to start one. A support group is not a substitute for individual therapy, and is not for everyone, but with the positive self-reports from participants and the growth of this approach to self-help, it is an option to be fully explored for the potential benefit to you, and also as an outlet for your giving to others.

STEPS YOU CAN TAKE TO ASSESS AND EXPAND YOUR SUPPORT SYSTEM:

- List your current sources of emotional support and consider whether any of them could be expanded, or if additions are indicated.

- List the people that you know who have chronic illnesses and ask a few of them where they seek emotional support.

- Check the appendix in the back of this book, the Department of Health in your community, and your local newspaper for information about available support groups.

- Discuss with your family the possibility of their attending a meeting of a family support group.

- Imagine, when you feel able, what kind of support you would like to offer to another person with your chronic illness.

NOTES

10

TAKING SOCIAL ACTION: YOU CAN MAKE A DIFFERENCE

Social action is a route out of the victim role. When people make a commitment to lighten the load of other chronically ill people, the mutual support they experience leads to strength and courage. Those who are willing to extend themselves to become involved in community action are people whose individual battles against illness haven't soured them on the possibilities and wonders of life.

When you help another, you are helping yourself. This is known as the "helper principle," i.e., that the helper gets as much help as the "helpee." Social or community action is a way to affirm yourself as you reach out to help others. Social action is not only therapeutic, but is powerful evidence that when people with common concerns get together and pool their knowledge and resources in the pursuit of a social goal, miracles can be accomplished. The oppressed, whether veterans of war, persons denied voting rights, or lacking accessibility to public amenities and civic/cultural resources, find strength and freedom from depression via social and political action.

Contributing money to a favorite program is a social action. Another option is writing a letter to a newspaper or a legislator in support of a pending law. You may choose from a wide range of activities, from relatively mild involvement to militant courses of action. The choices are yours. This chapter gives examples of different kinds of social action that you can take. They represent a small sample of the many options for improving the way society works so that people with chronic illness can have an easier time. These strategies involve designing unique service programs, legal efforts, original ways to raise public awareness, and dramatic protest rallies.

One example of a unique service program is Canine Companions for Independence. In this program dogs are trained as aides for ill people. The dogs wear blue and yellow bags, like saddle bags, to signify that they are graduates of the training center in Santa Rosa, California. It costs nearly seven thousand dollars to raise and train one of these dogs, and the money comes from donations. The dogs are raised by "foster parents" until they are seventeen months old.

A female retriever named Image is one of these dogs. She is a companion to Erek, a ninth-grader who suffers from muscular dystrophy and has never walked. With Image's assistance Erek can now take on new adventures such as shopping alone at malls. He has a helping hand--or paw--to push elevator buttons and take items off shelves for him. Store and restaurant employees are usually receptive to having the dog in their businesses. When they're not, Erek and Image flash cards that note their legal right to be in such establishments. Intense preparatory community effort went into providing this service.

Linda Galbraith who uses a wheel chair found her way of contributing to the community by compiling a resource guide of federal, state, and local aid for the handicapped. A militant protector of the rights of the disabled, she confronts able-bodied drivers who park in spaces reserved for the handicapped, sometimes slapping violators' cars with bumper stickers that read, "I'm not handicapped, but I parked here anyway."

Benjamin Mattlin chose to raise public consciousness by writing the following letter to a newspaper:

> As a person in a wheel-chair, I read with great interest the article on Physicist Stephen Hawking and his severe disability...I was disappointed, however, to see you refer to him as "confined to a wheelchair, a virtual prisoner in his own body." The expression "confined to a wheelchair," though common, is misleading and insulting. Wheelchairs are tools that enable us to get around. They are liberating, not confining. And as for his being a "prisoner in his own body." who is not?

A project that is close to Martha Rojas' heart is a support group of Mexican-American people suffering from diabetes. A diabetic herself, she wants to be in a position to help people deal with bi-cultural issues. It pains her that Hispanic families are reluctant to participate in health fairs, and that many Mexican-Americans are susceptible to the myths that are associated with diabetes. She knows people who believe that if you drink all of the lemon juice you can, it will make your blood sugar go down, that insulin will make you go blind, and that if you boil cactus and extract the juice (nopale), it will cure you. Her goal is to have a group that will provide both education and support for people with diabetes, people who have the complications that come with the disease, and who have language barriers as well. She will have cooking demonstrations, presentations from medical and nutritional experts, and use radio, other media and health fairs to reach out to reluctant potential participants. She wants to help them overcome their resistance to the medical and other help they need. It would be difficult to imagine a more effective role-model than Martha because of her charm, infectious enthusiasm, and dedication to her mission.

Amye Leong is also dedicated to a support group for those suffering from the same chronic illness that she has. Amye's foresight and positive attitude set the tone and mood for YET, a group for young people suffering from arthritis. She refers to it as "arthritis in prime time," and her program provides career planning, "fun rehabilitation techniques," information about joint replacements and other medical updates. Her New Year's greeting to the members read in part, "through your positive efforts, you have helped us prove that, collectively, we offer experience, resources, options and support in battling arthritis--just what the doctor ordered!"

Sonda Aronson has set up a support network which is not for sufferers of a particular illness, although she is severely disabled with allergies, asthma and chronic fatigue syndrome. Many substances trigger her asthma attacks. These include chemicals, natural substances and strong odors. This makes her daily life extremely limited. She has been print-handicapped for about four years. This means anything printed--books, magazines, newspapers--trigger asthma attacks. Despite these difficulties, she has achieved wide recognition for her work as an artist.

In 1985 Sonda started the Disabled Artists' Network.[1] Artists in this country face difficulties in financial support, promotion of their work, and the under-representation of women in galleries and museum shows. Physical disability compounds these problems, but Sonda is a problem-solver. Aware that chronically ill artists represent a wide variety of disabilities, and that these artists are involved in many different kinds of art, she established the Network as an information exchange and "living bulletin board" of disabled artists in the visual and sculptural arts. Part of the Network's program is focused on how artists can adapt their work methods to fit their disability.

Sonda is a woman of strong convictions. "The concept of 'overcoming,'" she states with conviction, "is the able-bodied way of trying to fit us into the status quo. If we fit into the status quo as is, society does not have to either change the way they see us or the way they think about us. We are usually viewed as 'different, weird,' or euphemized as 'special,' and this, of course, is idiotic nonsense. Able-bodied people have great difficulty seeing us as being much the same as them, with just some physical differences."

She believes that if society can see physically ill people as overcoming obstacles, no changes have to be made in the things that block their accessibility to society. If they are "overcoming" obstacles, or are "physically challenged" (she terms this another idiotic euphemism) society does not have to deal with their needs, especially the need for accessibility. She and other activists emphasize the need for wheel-chairs, ramps, curbcuts, public transportation and elevators, and so can you if you want to.

Sonda finds ways to work around her disabilities in order to create art, and also finds ways to create supportive networking for her fellow disabled artists. This is also an art--the art of living.

It is important that each person set his or her own goals and create his or her own path from victim to transcendence. Social action is one door that can open many others. Neil Marcus edits *Complete Elegance*, a 5000-circulation, Seattle-based publication for the disabled and puts out his own newsletter. Abbie Spellman, who was afraid to put her face in the water, started a program of swimming to raise money to end world hunger. Their profiles follow:

Neil Marcus: Fantastically Endowed Mime

Neil Marcus has not just devised a unique strategy to deal with his extreme physical handicap, he has found a way to capitalize on it with flair.

He has dystonia, a rare neurological disease that affects the coordination of muscles (they don't know why) and concerns the transmission of messages from the brain to the muscles. He has had it since he was a child. He talks and walks with extreme difficulty and spends much time in a wheel-chair. But he can stand

and walk alone in his fashion. Now he is thirty-four years old, and lives in Berkeley, California.

Besides editing *Complete Elegance*, he publishes *Special Effects*, a newsletter that focuses on issues of concern to disabled people. It reaches about 200 readers internationally, and addresses issues such as how companies and politicians can make life easier for people with physical limitations. Letters and inspirational writings by Marcus and others are included. Neil describes himself as a "fantastic spastic mime creatively endowed with disability." According to him, so-called "normality" is imaginary, it is a myth which is impossible to attain.

Neil is involved in political action for the disabled. One of his more dramatic forays into the social action arena occurred when he threw himself from his wheelchair onto the steps of a City Hall in 1982 protesting cutbacks in programs for helping physically impaired people.

The following is excerpted from a presentation he gave in 1986 on Personal Power and Disability:

*When you walk into a room full of people and there's a disabled person in that room, and she scares you or makes you want to avoid him, or she mystifies you, or you want to help but don't know how--when this happens, you are at the cutting edge of human liberation. Disabled Liberation is at the heart of all the oppression. Solve that one, and we're well on our way to a free society. See a disabled person clearly and chances are you'll be able to see yourself clearly. That is when there are no limits, and there **are** no limits as to when that will happen...*

*So where do you begin on this great move forward towards the ultimate liberation of peoples? I can sort of see that what I have done in **my** life has been a very effective first step. Making contact with lots of people. Helping them over hurdles that might have prevented them from getting to know me. Always reminding myself of my own worth and value. Presenting hope to people. (Life is precious* *regardless of the circumstances). Communicating the value of all kinds of life circumstances in writing. Communicating pride to people. And having a good life myself.*

What is hard is feeling that I am doing nothing. Feeling that my life is worthless. Not knowing what I want to do and feeling confused in general. However, I have just come up with the perfect contradiction to these feelings:

I have always worked hard to lead me and my people forward. Worked hard under the loneliest conditions with much confusion inside and surrounding me (disability-related). Every person who has had even the slightest contact with me has had their life changed in a very positive way and now it is time for me to recognize my own worth!

Neil is also a playwright. Access Theatre produces his *Storm Reading* in which he plays the leading role while his brother, Roger, a professional actor, speaks the lines. Those two young men, with the graceful Kathryn Voice signing the lines, form a compelling unit. There are biting parodies of the awkward, overbearing, cruel and patronizing approaches that people use when attempting to relate to people with physical problems. "How to approach me?" Neil's character asks. "If they would only look into themselves, they'd know. A good place to start is with a smile..."

Neil uses his whole self--the creative part, the humor, and the twisted body, in artistic expression that runs the gamut from dance to reflective satire about the roles of the physically impaired, and the non-physically impaired, in society.

Marcus' Father said of him that, "He makes (disabled people) feel like there's nothing stopping them." Lori Steinhauer of the Ventura Star Free Press wrote, "A viewing of *Storm Reading* reveals a man who has blazed a trail of adventure, fought for his belief and reached a gold mine of happiness that he does not want to hoard." Neil speaks little about his impairment and abhors attempts made by other people to tell how brave he is. "I'd rather emphasize something else, like my willingness to create vast social change," he says.

In *I Have a Voice,* Neil wrote,

> *I believe I have a voice. Words, feelings, observations; perceptions, thoughts. Thoughts that can move the world. I am a storm...When some people look at me they see only an autumn or winter...*

> *Some people, when they see my twisted frame, my dystonic disarray, embrace the storm. Their eyes light up, and they rush to hug me as a long-lost brother. As if embracing a storm was food for their soul.*

> *I can teach you to read a storm.*

Neil has the words, feelings, observations, perceptions and thoughts. Those attributes along with his love of life give him his remarkable voice.

Abbie Spellman: The Littlest Mermaid

Abbie Spellman has a rare hereditary disease called Freidrich's ataxia. It is a progressive degenerative illness which attacks the nervous system, causing an inability to coordinate voluntary muscle movements. When she was first told about the diagnosis, she learned that over time she might become blind or might have increased motor difficulties. She was told that she would be in a wheel-chair by the time she was twenty-two, but, she winks as she says, "I fooled them. I didn't have to use a wheel-chair until I was in my mid forties".

Abbie signed up for The Hunger Project in 1977 and became an "Ending Hunger Briefer" in 1983. She committed herself to swim one hundred miles in a year. She lines up sponsors who pledge certain amounts of money for each mile that she swims. The money is used toward combatting hunger. She keeps a record of the date, time, laps, and has each day's completed assignment signed by the person in charge of the pool. She swims for Project F.O.O.D. (Food Out of Donations), for a local hospice program, and for the Easter Seal Society Aquatics (Pool Therapy) Program. The Hunger Project is global with headquarters in New York. Abbie's goals go way beyond a strong sense of purpose--she has a mission.

Perhaps the most fantastic aspect of her swimming project is the fact that she made the commitment to it when she couldn't even swim, and was afraid to put her face in the water! She was talking with some children at a school for orthopedically handicapped children and felt challenged by them. She says they taught her to swim. "Children are good teachers," she says, "They know so much and are so wise. They teach you to love life. It's my vision for them to see that they can make a difference."

Swimming is not easy for Abbie because she doesn't have the use of her legs. She uses a backstroke most of the time, but then will flip over and take a few strokes that look like a combination of a crawl and a dog paddle while holding her breath. It takes a long time for her to dress and undress, and getting out of her wheel chair and into the pool is a feat in itself. She aims for 60 lengths a day, six days a week. It's a daily, four to five hour project.

When asked if being of service was one of the things that helps her cope with her chronic illness--is that "her secret"? Abbie answered "Isn't that the secret of life?" Sometimes she uses meditation, sometimes affirmations like, "I'm healthy and able and focused," "I am enjoying life," "I am serving myself and others," and "I am learning." She stresses that any learning helps you to be happy. When asked if her illness hadn't added some dimension to her philosophy, or if suffering hadn't strengthened her in some way, Abbie's response was that everybody has something, "Mine just happens to show."

Abbie, like a mermaid, seems more at home in the water than in the limelight. Some of the lines from Hans Christian's Anderson's *The Littlest Mermaid* fit. When she "...ventured to put her head up again, it looked as if all the stars were falling down to her from the sky..." "For you have the kindest heart of all." "And the daughters of the air said to the littlest mermaid, 'You have striven with your whole heart to do all the good that you can. By your sufferings, and by your courage in enduring them, you have raised yourself into the world and now you can gain an immortal soul....'" May the stars fall down on her--and may her vision that the rest of the world become committed, as she is committed to end world hunger, be realized. She is making a difference.

If writing plays or staging protest rallies are not your style, a good place to start is with the organization that is set up to help people with your illness. Consult them concerning their needs: for fund-raising, counseling, public education, or a speakers' bureau. When one of the authors of this book learned that her daughter had developed insulin-dependent diabetes, she made inquiries and found out that there is a need for diabetic children to be sent to summer camps that are structured for their special nutritional and exercise needs. Making a donation to the camp fee not only contributes to a child's life, but also is a gratifying experience for the donor. When you take action in the interest of a social cause of your choice, you can make a difference.

STEPS YOU CAN TAKE TO MAKE A DIFFERENCE:

- Think back to any volunteer work you have ever done that gave you pleasure. Consider whether there is any way you can apply those skills to a program for chronically ill people, or for people in need in other ways.

- Check the list of resources in the Appendix and the Yellow Pages for a health promotion organization of your choice. Make an inquiry as to their needs.

- Select an issue such as medical insurance, access to public transportation, or the training of animal aides and take a step toward becoming better informed about it. This step could be a call to the public library or a book store, or a question to your doctor or a community college.

- Remember that you make a social statement when you continue to do your heart's desire surmounting the constraints of your illness. Continue to write, paint, stay in school, write your congressmen. Find a way to continue your current interests, even if in a less active manner.

NOTES

11

CELEBRATING SMALL GAINS

Arnold Van Gennep's anthropological treatise, *The Rites of Passage,* published in 1908, describes the major transitions that occur throughout the cycle of life in primitive societies. They are childhood initiation rites, betrothal, marriage, pregnancy, childbirth, and going off to war. Each transition was treated as something that required an inner change where the old self was transformed into a new being with a new identity to fit his new outer social role. The trouble is that there are no prescribed rites of passage on the road map of the journey of the chronically ill--not for successful surgeries, or remissions, and certainly not for relapses, flare-ups, or the myriad set-backs that happen to the chronically ill that other people do not understand. Yet inner change and growth are called for, otherwise a cycle that is physical and downward will be accompanied by an inner emotional cycle that is also downward.

The challenge is to develop your own rites of passage, and this is not an easy task. When you feel yourself going down physically and know that you are getting worse, when there is no cure and you feel that you have lost all control over your life, this is a time for mourning your losses. You may feel like Dory Previn when she wrote:

> *i can't go on...*
> *i really*
> *can't go on*
> *i swear*
> *i can't go on*
> *so*
> *i guess*
> *i'll get up*
> *and go on*

You may be down physically, and you may have to be down emotionally for a while. But you don't have to stay there. To spiral upward spiritually, in spite of how rapidly you are spiralling downward physically, you can begin by focusing on what you have learned. Suffering, combined with reflective skills, can heighten awareness, and you are not the same person that you were at your last flare-up of symptoms. What have you learned about yourself? Your limitations? Your inner resources? The pluses and lacks in your support system? The nature of your disease?

After contemplating what you have learned, important questions for you to ask yourself are: What are my options? What would be a passive response to this new set of circumstances? An aggressive response? An assertive response? And which will I choose?

It is a process of moving from self-pity to self-forgiveness to self-acceptance and on to self-esteem. Self-esteem is the essential ingredient in a positive outlook. When it is possible again to see value in yourself, and in life, in spite of the unfair constraints imposed by your chronic illness, you're ready for the next set of questions which relate to what you have to be thankful for. There are always options and always things to be thankful for, and what you choose to believe is the most powerful option of all. More and more experts, including Norman Cousins, are discovering that the belief system can translate expectations into physiological change.

The power of expectation and the value of a positive attitude cannot be exaggerated. Michael F. Scheier, a psychologist at Carnegie-Mellon University in Pittsburgh, has found that optimists handle stress better than do pessimists. The power of expectation goes beyond mere achievement to visceral emotional qualities. "Our expectancies not only affect how we see reality but also affect the reality itself," according to Edward E. Jones, a psychologist at Princeton University who reviewed research on expectancy.

As you go through relapses, your life will not be the way it was before. However, it may have more profound meaning as you meet each new challenge in the course of your illness with your own version of a rite of passage. A rite of passage for growing through relapse involves in-depth questions as to where you are mentally and spiritually, and acknowledges the choices that you face, no matter how limited they may be. The most significant choices have to do with attitude, and if you cultivate a positive outlook, there are dividends in the growth of hope and in the possibility of self-fulfilling prophecies. The rite of passage that you devise should include the following three elements:

1. Acknowledgement of your growth.

2. Responsibility for your choices.

3. An optimistic attitude.

With such rites any physical spiraling downward will be more than balanced by a satisfying inner upsurge of spiritual growth.

Flare-ups and relapses, like all things in life, do pass. Remissions do occur and are cause for celebration for:

> *Rich the treasure,*
> *Sweet the pleasure--*
> *Sweet is pleasure after pain.*

John Dryden

Celebrations

It is good to celebrate yourself as a survivor, as a person with assets, and to implement your celebrations with rituals. We accept that milestones such as births, graduations, and weddings are occasions for gala observances, but with the misguided emphasis that our culture puts on modesty and humility, we overlook many marvelous opportunities to celebrate small successes. Other values also get in the way, such as the way we define success and honor bigness. However, in celebrating, tiny is often better.

The eminent composer and conductor, John Green, has a little ritual celebration in the form of a trademark, a carnation in his buttonhole, worn daily without fail. Green not only suffered a stroke that left him with impairments of speech and motion, but while fighting to recover, he fell and fractured a bone in his back. His trademark, the carnation, is his reminder that there is beauty in life and that we need to cherish and preserve it, and to create it if we can.

There is a place for big celebrations, of course. But big celebrations are less frequently called for and are easier to attain than the little daily rituals that improve the quality of life. Maximizing small successes is part of the art of living for everyone, not just the physically challenged. For example, the happy marriages are not the ones where the specialness of the relationship is recognized once or twice a year with an expensive gift. In happy marriages the partners exchange small strokes or "warm fuzzies" on an almost daily basis.

Wise therapists and effective parents know that picking up on small gains, giving them recognition, and building on them, is more effective than waiting for the "biggies" that may never happen. Celebrating the progression from a 'C' to a 'B' is a better strategy than waiting for an 'A.' And there is always **something** to celebrate even if it's a triviality, like the dog's birthday.

If you cannot think of anything else to celebrate at the moment, celebrate your survivorship. You not only are a survivor, but you take initiative in seeking help. Witness your reading this book. Congratulate yourself and start thinking of ways to celebrate. The last page of *How to Survive the Loss of a Love*, reads:

> *I loved,*
> *Which was purgatory.*
>
> *I lost,*
> *Which was hell.*
>
> *And I survived.*
> *Heaven!*[1]

So whatever your particular purgatory, or your special hell, you have survived, and you deserve a celebration ceremony.

A celebration is a form of self-recognition. Theodore Isaac Rubin in *Compassion and Self-Hate: An Alternative to Despair*[2] wrote:

"Our society in its confusion over the value of modesty puts too little importance on the process of self-recognition. If we take ourselves with enough appropriate and appreciative seriousness, this dilutes the compulsive and frustrating need for recognition from others. Self-recognition involves extensive knowledge and acceptance of one's assets and the ready ability to tap and use them in one's own behalf. This is the antithesis of feelings of inadequacy that lead to either self-effacing compliance or compensatory grandiosity."

Rituals are ways to claim and savor your gains, to translate such self-recognition into action, to affirm it.

Alexandra Stoddard provides specific ways in which to apply this philosophy. Her charming book, *Living a Beautiful Life: Five Hundred Ways to Add Elegance, Order, Beauty and Joy to Every Day of Your Life*,[3] explains that by "paying careful attention to the simple details of daily tasks and to our immediate surroundings we can live vitally and beautifully all the days of our lives. It takes a commitment to enjoy each day fully." "Rituals" is her term for patterns you create in your everyday living that uplift the way you do ordinary things, so that a simple task rises to the level of something special, ceremonial, ritualistic. She goes on to assert that, "Rituals can elevate the way you feel about yourself, your life, and make you more peaceful and more free, more useful to others." She adds that, "Pleasing details change the things we do into activities that celebrate being alive, and that shore us up for the rigors of life." With the added effort that you, as a chronically ill person, have to exert to get through your days, it can be a worthy challenge to design rituals that will, "shore (you) up for the rigors of (your) life. Rituals bring warmth and comfort; they give you things to count on enjoying every day."

The recommended place to start is with stimulating your senses, so first do an inventory of what pleases your senses. If you answer the following questions fully, with adequate experimentation and testing, you will have completed an in-depth exercise in self-awareness:

1. What colors make you feel good?

2. What fragrances make you feel good?

3. What music makes you feel good?

4. What foods and beverages make you feel good?

5. What textures do you enjoy touching?

The possibilities for designing rituals that introduce more sensual pleasures into your daily or weekly routine are endless. Following are examples of how four chronically ill people created rituals and celebrations to enhance their lives.

Perry

For years Perry looked forward to puttering in his vegetable garden in his free time, but he had to quit active gardening because of severe arthritis. He went through a period of grieving since this was a major loss to him. His vegetables had been his pride and joy. He turned his back on the yard and quoted Charles Dudley Warner with some bitterness, "What a man needs in gardening is a cast-iron back, with a hinge in it."

After several months Perry hired a gardener and restructured the garden to reduce painful maintenance chores. He reluctantly replaced the rustic but uncomfortable furniture and picturesque stone bench with well constructed chairs with thick, sturdy cushions. A new stone wall cut down and redefined the space to more workable proportions. Waist-high planters provided work areas that did not require bending.

Now Perry, with help, has achieved a new kind of garden with fewer vegetables and more flowers. He is flourishing with them. Each evening he puts on his old Harvard sweat shirt with a hood, enjoying its fleecy feel, its warmth, and the pleasant associations with the past that it evokes. He walks the small circumference of his garden conscious of how the gentle exercise is helping his tired muscles and sore joints. He savors the sweet scent of jasmine and its white starlike shapes against its dark, shiny green leaves. He enjoys the sounds of the birds chirping, and is contemplating getting a fountain to have the sound of splashing water. He relishes a few bites of Triscuits before tossing the remains to the birds.

For quite a long time, Perry minded that his garden was changed so much. But now he takes pleasure in it, and in his ceremonial walks around it. He has gone back to quoting Charles Dudley Warner but now it's, "No man but feels more of a man in the world if he have a bit of ground that he can call his own. However small it is on the surface, it is four thousand miles deep, and that is a very handsome property." Occasionally Perry holds a larger celebration in the form of a garden party, but the daily, small, ritualistic celebrations of having found a way to continue to enjoy his garden are the most meaningful to him.

Melissa

Melissa doesn't have a garden, though she does tend potted plants. She also has lupus. She comes home from work completely drained, but instead of rifling through her mail and flopping down in front of the T.V. she has a winding-down ritual that she revels in. First she heats water for tea, selecting the flavor with care, then she gets into her most comfortable clothes; jeans and moccasins, puts on a Joni Mitchell record, and settles on the couch with the mail, the newspaper, a fine, hand-tooled leather notebook and a fat purple pen. She listens to her answering machine, reads her mail, marks the program(s) in the T.V. guide that might interest her, reads the paper and jots down in her notebook experiences of the day that she wants to remember. It's her time to celebrate that she's made it through the day and that she's home again. She reviews her day and plans her evening, but the drift of this winding-down time is to savor the taste and aroma of the herb tea, the ambiance of her cozy den, the sound of a soothing voice singing favorite songs, the feel of fine leather, the color purple on shiny white paper--all sensual pleasures in the present. The closing ritual to this reverie is the tending of a plant or two that need TLC.

Jenny

With Jenny it's a bathing ritual, and she makes a production as well as a ceremony out of it. She is one of the estimated eighty million Americans who suffer from back pain. Jenny would like to have a spa with jets to help relieve the pain, but she compensates for that lack with other accouterments. A friend painted three walls of her bathroom sea-green with waving aquatic plants and large fish swimming around. The faces of the fish and an otter bear suspicious resemblances to members of Jenny's family, her doctor, and some of her friends.

The mirrored wall reflects billowing curtains made of a seaweed-like fabric. These and the oceanic murals create an undulating, underwater effect. Jenny has an inflated rubber pillow, and her "bathtub toys" are a floating tray that holds a glass and a book. Her radio, cordless phone, water proof clock and luxuriant robes and towels complete the picture. This makes it easier for Jenny to extend her heated bath to the recommended time without getting bored. It's less expensive and more to her taste than massage, and she enjoys figuring out how to stimulate all of her senses--smell (bath salts and soap), sight (sea shells, colorful towels), taste (juice in her floating coaster), sound (radio), and feeling (bath oils, rubdown). Even her sense of humor is tickled with the murals made of caricatures and the incongruity, to her, of her ritualistic, solitary celebrations in her bathtub. But she continues to acknowledge her small successes in dealing with her pain. She believes these observances are an alternative to brooding, self-pity and depression.

Margo

Margo was an interpretive dancer until multiple diseases damaged her body to the extent that she had to quit. She greets the dawn with highly stylized, graceful bodily movements as she gives thanks for having lived through the night, no matter how difficult a night it was, and gives thanks for the new day. She then practices her own brand of Yoga that she developed in consultation with her Yoga instructor and a physical therapist. The next step in her lengthy morning ritual is deep meditation. She chooses her mantra with care, a hibiscus blossom, an unusual stone, a piece of fruit, or a lighted sand candle. She feels that after her close brushes with death, celebrations of life are in order and that they develop her spiritual nature. She uses meditation to find answers to questions, knowing that the answers come from deep inside her subconscious. After these exercises in contemplation, Margo turns to her journal. She records whatever parts of her dreams that she can remember, insights gained from her meditation, and goals for the day.

Margo then bathes, dresses, and applies make-up so painstakingly that these steps, too, are ritualistic. Finally, the crossword puzzle, breakfast, a second cup of decaffeinated coffee, and she is ready for her day. Before she began these rituals she stayed in bed all day more often than not, railing at the fate that left her so disabled. She believes that her idiosyncratic manner of celebrating life, beginning in the morning, works for her but that everyone needs to design his or her own special way.

You may have a garden ritual, a winding-down ritual, a bath ritual, a morning ritual for beginning your day, or something entirely different. Design celebrations of your successes, no matter how small, and design them to meet your special needs and tastes. Use them as a pleasant goal, to counter depression, help you live in the present, and enhance the quality of your life.

STEPS YOU CAN TAKE TO CELEBRATE SMALL GAINS:

- List some reasons to celebrate: your survival, small successes achieved by you, a member of your family, or a friend.

- Congratulate yourself out loud for one of your successes, tell some one about it, and record it in your journal.

- Identify your favorite color, fragrance, kind of music, food, beverage, and texture and enjoy indulging these tastes.

- Plan a celebration and design a ritual to meet your special needs and tastes. This may be just for your own pleasure, or you may want to include friends.

NOTES

PART III

LIVING AT YOUR PERSONAL BEST

This section chronicles the changes a person experiences as she or he moves from being a victim of a disease, to a survivor, to one whose identity transcends a particular physical condition. Ingredients are identified that give you the satisfaction of living at your personal best with a chronic condition.

Turning points are those events, intuitions, and choices that lead to change and get you on the road toward living at your personal best. Getting rid of attitudes and beliefs that are no longer useful can be a new beginning to getting on with your life. Some useful perspectives toward this end are discussed in Part III. Living at your personal best, so that you can soar, like the phoenix, up and beyond your earlier sense of self, often brings you to an encounter with questions of spirituality. First you question, then you heal, as several examples of people's lives will illustrate.

It may surprise you that the traits that facilitate transcendence are not singular, but that the key to moving beyond survivorship is balance. The final chapter includes a guide to assessing where **you** are in relation to living a balanced life and transcending pain.

ARTISTRY

Life is a painting my friend
With no beginning or end
It's just a process in time
Where shadows appear to be lines
You choose all the colors and tones
You're never painting alone
And when you paint from the heart
Your life is a work of art[1]

Sharon Riddell

12

IDENTIFYING TURNING POINTS

Turning points are those forks in the road at which decisions and commitments are made. They may be clear at the time, or only appear to be clearly decisive points in retrospect. They may grow out of a rational process, such as the building of a skill that helps you cope, or from an intuitive flash of insight. Turning points may occur several times during the course of a chronic illness. They move you from being a victim to being a survivor, to becoming a person whose life transcends the confines of disease. By learning to identify turning points you can better recognize your growth forward.

Marsha, 31, was bedridden for six months when she came to a decision, or a turning point, in her life. While looking at the four walls of her bedroom she saw three choices: she could commit suicide (thereby becoming a victim of her circumstances), accept what came her way (surviving in spite of it all), or fight, asking herself the hard question, "Who am I now?" Fortunately, she remembered her mother's saying that her very first words as a tiny girl were, "Me do it!" Marsha said to herself: "This is not going to rob me of my life." Consistent with Victor Frankl's concept of depression, she was about to begin the journey out of meaninglessness, to affirm life despite suffering. She was making choices about attitude.

Turning points, or crisis points, compel a struggle between the need for security and the challenge of risk. The Chinese symbol for crisis is comprised of two characters, one translating into risk, the other into opportunity. In order to move into this place of opportunity, you must confront your worst fears. Some common fears that chronically ill people have are:[1]

"Becoming a bag lady."

"Being dependent on others."

"That my arms will give out and I will drop my baby."

"Dying before I've had a full enough life."

"That my energy will give out and my disease will get worse."

"An unbearable future that I won't know how to deal with."

These fears represent self-concepts and expectations, and refer to the future, not the present.

In chronic illness, change often comes not by choice, but by what sociologist, Gordon Allport refers to as "the power of the fait accompli," or by chance. You are drafted into change; you have no choice. Initially there is great resistance to change. You scramble to protect the investment you have in relationships and roles. It is quite natural to react as a victim at this stage. A turning point occurs when there is a change in attitude, when you leave the victim stage for that of a survivor.

Changes in Attitude: A Mental Housecleaning

Sometimes the degree of physical and mental pain you suffer suggests that your attitudes and beliefs are no longer useful. You begin to sort these out, keeping some, but letting go of others. This sorting out, or mental housecleaning, is part of a process of restoration. Like an old house that is being pared to the bone and restored, you are seeking the authentic parts of yourself that will become the base for the quality life you want. Part of this sorting involves looking at the mythical thinking that surrounds chronic illness.

Myths are beliefs or accounts unfounded in fact. They serve the purpose of explaining the nature of an event. They can be useful or not. When you're anxious, it is natural to look for cause-and-effect relationships and to regress to a more childlike emotional state. Illness is apt to make you feel more dependent and more prone to self-blame and regrets. You may feel guilty for enjoying some of the attention that you receive. You may find yourself thinking:

"I always suspected that I was weak and dependent"

"I feel like I'm being punished in some way"

This is negative mythical thinking.

You may have outgrown this kind of self-blame but there are contemporary myths, too. With the recent emphasis on holistic health, and the role that emotions play, there is an implication that you caused your physical problems by not thinking the "right" thoughts. You may assume that your capacity to fantasize helpfully is limited, or that you have somehow brought on your illness, perhaps by worrying too much. This is also mythical thinking.

A New Collection of Attitudes That Work

The process of exploding and countering myths can look like this:

ATTITUDE REASSESSMENT

OUTWORN MYTH	NEW VALUE
(Useless Belief)	(Useful Belief)
Independence is an essential goal.	Interdependence is a goal that I aspire to.
To be inactive is to be useless.	To be active is to do; to be inactive is to **be**. I honor both.
To be physically disabled is to be asexual	My sexuality expresses my sense of wholeness; the physical, emotional, and social aspects that express my maleness or femaleness.
Everyone is healthy except me.	Everyone has their healthy and unhealthy times including me.

How can you counter faulty inner assumptions?

The clue that leads to the unmasking of outworn myths is the word, "should." Do you feel that you "should not" have these feelings? You can have these universal feelings without acting on them, and sometimes you can use them as topics for good communication with members of your family.

Are you feeling that you "should" try to ignore pain because showing or even acknowledging suffering will indicate weakness? Do you try to ignore the whole subject of your illness in the hope that it will go away? Do you believe that paying attention to pain somehow feeds it? If so, you are not alone. No one can be objective about her own emotional involvement with her own body. Feeling weak and dependent for a day, or a month does not mean you are a weak and dependent person. Bringing your mythical thinking to your conscious awareness, and examining it, is a step toward attaining a healthy perspective.

This process takes time, insight, and new learning on a continuing basis. But exploding your myths is worth the effort for the process helps resolve the grief and pain that result from faulty thinking. It has been said that unresolved grief is the biggest clinical problem of our age. By rethinking your beliefs and attitudes you can reach a turning point in coping successfully with your condition.

Identifiable Turning Points

You have reached a turning point in your personal growth when you:

- Feel yourself moving through the grief of losses.
- No longer feel like a victim.
- Can begin to problem solve.
- Recognize your options.
- Have adjusted your attitudes and beliefs to your current life style.
- Can identify positives.
- Have energy to give to others.

Two modern psychologies offer a way of thinking that supports a new attitude. **Rational Emotive Therapy**, developed by Dr. Albert Ellis is one of them. Eric Bern's **Transactional Analysis** is the other.

Rational Emotive Therapy[2]

Rational Emotive Therapy entails using your rational mind to counter emotion-laden feelings. It requires that you take responsibility for, or "own" your thoughts instead of blaming others. A step in this direction is to say "I feel (think, did)" rather than "You make me..." It means translating a negative sensation into a thought. For example, "I feel angry and sad when you talk around me just because I am in a wheel-chair."

Emotion-laden feelings support the old beliefs. They provide irrational thoughts full of "shoulds," and "musts." They support wishful thinking and unrealistic goals that embody the old attitudes such as, "I must not let my family down, even though I have fatigue and pain." These attitudes lead to self-defeating behavior, because as much as you may want to fulfill this wish, your body may not be able to cooperate. The beginning of being able to be there for another, is to be there for yourself.

Here are some rational, realistic attitudes that lead to new beliefs about yourself and others:

- I would prefer to feel great today, but I can accept the fact that I don't.

- Keeping the house clean is definitely a desirable thing to do, but I can be satisfied with a less-than-perfect standard.

- It's really nice to have the love and approval of my family and friends, but I can find pleasure in my own acceptance of myself.

- I want to be "my old self" again, but I recognize that I have adjustments to make so that I can be happy. And the new self that is emerging will be valuable and useful to me.

Out with old self-defeating ideas, traits, and activities! In with an accepting attitude born of liking yourself as you are. It is a process of working on yourself as you grieve the self that is no more. What you tell yourself has impact on how you feel, so delete the "shoulds", "musts," and "ain't it awfuls." Replace those self-defeating words that keep you stuck in a victim role with, "wants," "prefers," and "it would be nice if." "Awfulizing" creates a melodrama of your life. When you find yourself starring in your own melodrama, at least find some humor in it!

Transactional Analysis (TA)[3]

The Transactional Analysis approach can help you understand how you think, feel, and most importantly, communicate. To think differently about your life situation can result in a turning point in attitude and relationships. The premise is that every one needs "strokes" and designs a "life script" and plays "games" based upon early beliefs, probably developed in childhood. TA suggests the presence of three active "ego states" that are dynamic and observable. The ego states are:

PARENT (P)——————— Critical and Controlling or Nurturing and Growth Promoting

ADULT (A)——————— Absorbs information, stores and retrieves it; is rational, logical and a good problem solver

CHILD (C)——————— Creative, Intuitive, or Rebelious, Conforming.

Each person communicates from one or another of these ego states in conversations within himself and with others. It is not fair to say that one is right and another wrong. It is more useful to say that each level of response fits a particular stage of coping. When your sense of self is threatened, an inner dialogue may go something like this:

C (CHILD): "I'm scared I don't know what to expect. Someone please take care of me!"

A (ADULT): "Don't worry. I will find out everything I can about what causes this...and what we can do about it."

C (CHILD): "Maybe if I ignore it, it will go away."

CP (Critical Parent): "Humm...I wonder what you did to cause this? Was it the way you let all those things pile up and create stress? You know what they say about people like you these days."

A (ADULT): "Now you know that's irrational. You sound like you think you're being punished. You are not a bad person. We'll learn how to cope. I will read, study, talk with others, get good medical advice..."

NP (NURTURING PARENT): "And I will comfort you, and love you always..."

C (CHILD): "Tell me that...over and over again..."

The task is to activate the ego states of the adult who uses information to recognize options, and the nurturing parent who always accepts and loves the scared child within. By strengthening these two ego states, your critical parent side will shrivel up and die like the wicked witch of the east in the *Wizard of Oz*. You will bring comfort to your inner scared child, identify the positives in your situation, and encourage that intuitive, creative, child of the spirit.

Intuition and Turning Points

Intuition is that hunch you get, that sense that something is right or wrong. Your intuition can lead you to **know** that a change is needed. Marsha's intuition led her to the point where her attitude about herself was brought into question. It led her back in her memory to her first words of "Me do it!" You will strengthen your intuition by cultivating reflective skills (Chapter 8). Combining intuition and analytical skills moves you towards adjusting your attitudes and beliefs to your current life style so you can live at your personal best. An example of some one who has achieved this is Pam.

Pam: No Pedestals

Pam knows it is not just the attitudes of the chronically ill that must be adjusted. Stress can come from people who want to put you on a pedestal, make you different, even "better." To her it is almost as bad to be put on a pedestal as it is to be locked in a closet. It's just as separating. Pam had polio when she was four years old and now suffers with post polio syndrome. One of her legs is partially paralyzed, while the other is completely paralyzed. "Putting us on a pedestal is saying that we are different. It is insidiously dangerous to the average person, and we are average people," says Pam. She is concerned about what she calls the "media blitz." "Role-modeling can work both ways. Skiing down the slopes on one leg or crossing the country in a wheel-chair can inspire or defeat, depending on the ego strengths of the reader. Fantastic successes, if they contrast with your life, can generate anxiety or even guilt."

If Pam has a strong aversion to pedestals, she has an even stronger aversion to stereotypes. She explains that some physically impaired people are not doing well, are even failing in many areas. Others are achieving wonderful feats. "The rest of us are right in the middle, i.e. average," she adds. It is a little hard to perceive of Pam as "average" because she comes across as such a competent, confident career woman. She is a social worker specializing in work with the mentally retarded, now called the developmentally disabled.

There are many issues that you have to deal with, Pam goes on to explain. A year ago she kept hitting "that wall of fatigue" to the point where she was forced to consider going from crutches to wheel-chair--first for big trips, then for little trips, then for her housework, and finally for all of the time. It got so that facing a staircase could strike terror in her heart, and to resist any longer would be to take the enormous risk of losing the strength of her upper body. If you break a wrist when you don't have the use of your legs you're in real trouble. Pam had a difficult time functioning both at home and at work. She broke up tasks by thinking, "If I can just get to the lobby (of her office building), then, "If I can just make it to the elevator," then, "Now, if I can only get to the receptionist's desk," and then, "If I can just make it to my own office." She had to stay focused on just getting through the day.

It was a long period for Pam from crutches to wheel-chair. "Grief comes in waves as we move through life stages," she comments.

When asked about post polio syndrome Pam said, "It's just like coming down with it all over again--a new disease, a 'kicker,' it's not fair. We dealt with it once and now we have to deal with it all over again. My muscles wore out." In going to the wheel-chair there was more loss, more grieving, more adjusting, and an inevitable period of depression.

It is a turning point for an individual or a family when positives can be identified. It is a sign that the adjustment is being handled, and that the person once more has gained some sense of control. Pam found that she is not as fatigued. She can carry her own packages, and she doesn't have to face the terrible fear of falling. There is no loss of dignity in the way she zips around in her wheel-chair. Assertiveness and graciousness are combined in the way she deals with colleagues and clients alike. She can still use crutches on rare occasions, and she is so experienced she can look at others on crutches and give accurate and wry estimates as to how long they've been using them.

Pam may describe herself as average, but she has the strength and authenticity to be herself, and that self is unique. Her response would probably be, "But then, so are we all," her way of staying off a pedestal. She may not choose to call herself a role model, but her struggle is productive of insight and skill in itself--witness the work that she is committed to and the perspective that she has developed. She can look back and identify turning points where she recognized options and found the energy to give to others.

As you adapt to and understand your chronic illness you can recognize certain qualities that describe different stages of coping. The following chart will help you clarify where you are in the progression from victim to survivor to transcender:

GROWTH TOWARD TRANSCENDENT RESPONSES

	VICTIM	SURVIVOR	TRANSCENDER
ATTITUDE:	Feels has no choice. Trapped.	Can use some skill to go on. Resigned.	Cuts through fear. Works through depression. Writes personal life script.
ENERGY USED FOR:	Resistance to change. Fear. Passivity.	Maintaining in the face of change.	Assimilating change. Growth.
QUESTIONS:	Why me?	What do I need to do?	Who am I? What can I do? What do I want to do?
LEVEL OF RISK:	Low. Seeks the security of the known.	Low-medium. Seeks to establish and maintain comfort.	High. Tolerates discomfort for the sake of growth.

STEPS YOU CAN TAKE TO IDENTIFY TURNING POINTS IN YOUR LIFE:

- Be aware of the "shoulds" that you say to yourself. Analyze whether they are the basis of myths or self-defeating thoughts. Counter them with new and more useful beliefs.

- Recognize and analyze situations where you are in your parent-ego state, your adult-ego state, and your child-ego state. Assess whether there are any changes you want to make in your style of communicating.

- Refer to the **Growth Toward Transcendent Responses** chart and identity moves you have made, backward and forward, in your path toward transcendence.

13

SPIRITUALITY AND ITS HEALING POWER

T he life of the spirit can be called the life of the larger self. The spirit is both deep inside, and expands to include all of life. Laura Chester, in her book *Lupus Novice*,[1] which relates her struggle with a diagnosis of lupus, writes, "No matter how the spiritual is met or rejected, it suddenly seems to rise up as a route, the golden road, out of illness, away from the physical body, or a way to meet the deepest part of the body, the untouchable source."

During the period of time that chronically ill persons were interviewed for this book, these men and women in the trenches suffering said, "You can't talk about living with chronic illness without talking about spirituality."

This chapter discusses the healing power that can be found when you listen to your intuition and practice the disciplines required of spiritual life. As people experience the life of the spirit in different ways, examples follow of how chronic illness led four people to develop their spirituality.

Val

At age 30 as a young wife and mother, Val contracted polio. Later in life during a six year period she was diagnosed with cancer and had a mastectomy, suffered a stroke which paralyzed her left side, and grieved the premature death of her son from an industrial accident. These events challenged the once strong faith of a very logical woman who needed everything to make sense. She said:

> *My breast was gone, the limbs on the left side of my body had a mind of their own, my beloved son had been taken, and I cried out as did Jesus on the cross, 'Father, why have you forsaken me?' God was gone, there was nothing except me and this world. All of the things that I had always been able to do, like walk on the beach and let out screams and yells in my private places, all that was taken.*

Val followed her intuition. She reached down deep inside to draw upon skills and resources she had never needed before. She goes on:

> *I had to find something to fill that emptiness or go absolutely insane. I began to read. I drew on everything I had ever learned, and put everything I ever knew together from my own theology. I began to read from Hinduism, Islam, and Zen. I read Joseph Campbell's **The Power of Myth**, and re-read William Buckley's interview with Malcom Muggeridge. I underlined the words, 'The approach to God is through the acceptance of a mystery.' Well, I sure couldn't understand why all of these things had happened to me, so that must qualify!*

> *All of this put underpinnings under the child-like faith I'd had.*

That was not the end of it for Val. One day a friend told her she must have sinned. "You are praying wrong, and God has deserted you," said her friend. Betrayal of a friend's trust was heaped upon despair.

180

I sat down in a chair and prayed desperately, which was to pray simplistically, out of need. All of a sudden this horrible weight I'd felt on me began to lift. There was nothing magical, just a slow lifting of this horrible weight. That was my miracle, and the first sign I had that God was down deep inside me. I sat in the chair and let it happen over about one-half hour.

Val is able to say with a sparkle in her eye that the magic is in reaching down deep inside to find her strength, and she now has what she calls the "nerve to know truth as it is given."

Barbara

One winter day Barbara took a nasty fall on the ice near her office. She was a newly single woman in her early 40s who had been active on the tennis courts, upwardly mobile in her career, and proud of being in control of her life. Muscles in her upper back were badly twisted, pain radiated through her shoulders, up into her neck, then back down the middle of her back. Prognosis for recovery was six weeks. Two and a half years later she lives with myofascial pain, or pain that continues beyond the original healing. When it began, standard physical therapy had little effect. Pain pills and the heating pad provided only monentary relief. Stretch classes, bio-feedback, massage and reconditioning exercises followed. Barbara got better for periods of time, but she did not get well.

It wasn't until she addressed a lifelong depression by entering psychotherapy that she began to see that emotional healing was tied to physical healing. She said, "My injury was a metaphor; this was a package deal. My progress, physically was tied to emotional and spiritual healing." Pain was the teacher. It was the one thing she could not control. By examining her life she saw that she had been ruled by fear and a need to be in control. She had become afraid of change, alienated from people, and felt unimportant.

Barbara's pain was more than physical--it was emotional and spiritual. Now, three years later, she says:

I view my back problem as a gift. I am in better psychological health. This has been an experience of a rebirth on a spiritual dimension that has enabled me to develop a sense of self that is internal, versus external. As I have let go of always needing to be in control, there is a positive response from people around me to the person that I am, in fact, becoming. This whole experience has been a trauma of large proportion, out of which I am developing strength. I feel on the verge of a new life; my vision has opened on horizons never known before. My ability to be in touch with my subconscious is instrumental in giving me the guidance I need to deal with my life and feelings.

Barbara finds that the disciplines for physical healing are the same as those necessary for spiritual healing: time, meditation, an open, receptive attitude, imagery, and patience. She is incorporating these skills and disciplines into her lifestyle. She is receiving a spiritual gift out of her suffering.

Richard

Richard was a free-spirited student at a large university in the 1960s. While pursuing the academic life he joined a meditation group. Life in the ivory tower soon palled and he left to join a religious community. That also lost its appeal and he returned to the city to work. It was while programming computers that he developed diabetes. Fear gripped his soul, for he had seen his father struggle with the frustrations of being a "brittle" case, unable to keep his blood sugars in a manageable range. But the 1980s are different, and so is Richard. His computer-like mind looks at monitoring blood sugars as a challenge; he is interested in improving the technology. In fact, he is talking with a buddy who works in the bio-medical technology field about collaborating to improve the state-of-the-art in this fast growing field. A bonus for Richard is that he is able to look at the precision of blood testing, and the necessity to rest, exercise, keep his stress level low, and eat correctly as a kind of spiritual discipline. It has given him a focus for both his meditation and his work. He experiences himself as a more spiritually aware person than he once was. He still gets frustrated about the constant need for self discipline, and he occasionally "loses it," as he puts it, but on good days, which are most of them, he knows the management of diabetes has brought discipline, focus, and structure into his life, which is what he sought in spiritual life in his student days. "It has matured me," he says.

Elsa

Diabetes is different for Elsa whose profile is in Chapter 8 on reflective skills. There has been no predictable path to good management. A diagnosis in childhood combined with the nature of her own metabolism and the technology available 25 years ago resulted in an experience similar to being on the end of the line in the childhood game of crack-the-whip. There was no predictable sense of control. Elsa finds most "How to" approaches are predicated on being in control, and that doesn't work for her. Physical crises become spiritual crises. When her vision is threatened she wants more than lessons on how to read braille. "Extreme stress opens one to the larger questions of life," she says.

Stress has challenged Elsa to become an explorer. Her spiritual healing comes from a broad spectrum of sources, Jungian psychology and dream work, the study of American Indian culture with its symbol of the bear as the Great Mother who comforts and heals, and her strong Christian faith.

Before Elsa understood anything about intuition, she found her private prayers, or "long conversations with God," dovetailed with events in her life. One week she challenged God to show her that he existed and cared. She visited her parents' church and said

My heart sank when I saw the sermon was from the book of Daniel. How could that possibly help me? Then the minister said he'd had another sermon planned that week but had been called to change his message, knowing that there were people in the congregation who were facing difficult times. He wanted us to know that Christ would be with us, too, just as he had been with three captive Israelites who were thrown in the fiery furnace when they refused to serve false gods. He went on to base his sermon on Daniel 1: 13-27

Elsa continues to be curious and receptive. She says, "I have found in my woundedness the path to wholeness. This does not imply it is the only path; generalities cannot be made. Each person responds differently and must find his own unique way to handle his problem."

Finding Your Own Way

When your life is governed to a greater or lesser extent by chronic illness, choices are made, and life gets reprioritized. You may have less reliability on physical energy. You may find that you mature at a faster rate than your peers. Quietly at first, and then with skill and choice, you begin to develop mental, emotional, and spiritual aspects of yourself.

Like Richard and Barbara, you may find the disciplines of treatment become spiritual disciplines, and hence, steps toward transcendence. Like Val and Elsa, you may find your earlier faith challenged, explored, and then expanded. Both women reassessed their old beliefs to find what works for them now, as they cope daily with chronic illness. The crisis of faith and restoration of Self, often follows a pattern:

1. Pre-crisis: familiar coping skills and faith.

2. Crisis: diagnosis or change in condition.

3. Anxiety, depression, and pain: feeling betrayed.

4. Allowing yourself to be open to new experience.

5. Reconstructing a faith out of experience (all of who you are helps this to happen: your skills, your support systems, your strengths).

6. Restored sense of Self.

Your resources are vast--from quiet reflective writing and thinking, to family, friends and community--in which to explore questions of faith. You may find a part of your spiritual healing comes from giving back to others. Service as a pathway to healing the spirit is a component of the world's great religions.

The way to authenticity is the way from victim through mere survival to the spiritual energy of transcendence.

STEPS YOU CAN TAKE TO DEEPEN YOUR SPIRITUALITY AND HEALING POWER

- Reread your journal, the chapter on cultivating your reflective skills, and some spiritual writings which appeal to you.

- Take time to sort out your spiritually healing attitudes from those that are not useful.

- Consult clergy, friends, or family as you feel inclined, but also keep your own counsel.

- Review the "Steps You Can Take" at the end of each chapter. Congratulate yourself for the ones you have taken, and decide which ones you want to complete or repeat.

- Make your own list of steps to take to further deepen your spirituality, to live creatively with your chronic illness, and to transcend the pain.

14

SOARING TO GREAT HEIGHTS

What are the traits that facilitate transcendence? Many books list qualities for living optimally. For example, Dr. Bernie Siegel, in his powerful and inspiring book, *Love, Medicine and Miracles: Lessons Learned About Self-Healing from a Surgeon's Experience with Exceptional Patients,*[1] eloquently explores the link between mind and body and discusses traits that help you to become exceptional.

In Dr. Siegel's book he also tells of Dr. Kenneth Pelletier who made a psychological study of patients who recovered despite great odds. He found five characteristics common to all of them:

1. Profound intrapsychic change through meditation, prayer, or other spiritual practice.

2. Profound interpersonal changes. As a result of spiritual changes their relations with other people had been placed on a more solid footing.

3. Alterations in diet: These people no longer took their food for granted. They chose their food carefully for optimum nutrition.

4. A deep sense of the spiritual as well as material aspects of life.

5. A feeling that their recovery was not a gift nor spontaneous remission, but rather a long, hard struggle that they had won for themselves.

Six characteristics mark optimal performers, says Charles A. Garfield, a performance psychologist. These people are able to transcend their previous levels of accomplishment. They avoid the so-called comfort zone, that no-man's land where a person feels complacent. They do what they do for the art of it and guided by compelling, internal goals. They solve problems rather than place blame. They confidently take risks after laying out the worst consequences beforehand, and they are able to rehearse coming actions or events mentally. None of these characteristics are dependent on an intact body.

None of these lists is exhaustive, nor is the one that follows, but it may point the way toward a winning attitude and be a guide toward transcendence. This list of traits will help you keep perspective. Perspective in relation to chronic illness means keeping a balance between grieving the losses that come with chronic illness, and using remaining capabilities to live as full a life as possible. It means a stable balance between feeling and fact, "right brain/left brain," and concern for self and concern for others. These and other pairs of complementary traits have to be kept in balance to maintain perspective. Our assets, if taken to extremes, become our liabilities. That is why lists of desirable singular characteristics can seem simplistic and, in come cases, even contradictory. So what are the traits that facilitate transcendence?

BALANCED TRAITS

PERSPECTIVE

Independence _____ Dependence

Acceptance _____ Constructive Rebellion

Solitude _____ Sociability

Seriousness _____ Humor

Purposefulness _____ Flexibility

Planfulnesss _____ Spontaneity

Self-care _____ Concern For Others

Positive Self-image _____ Positive Image Of Others

Faith And Trust _____ Healthy Skepticism

Toughness _____ Accommodation

PERSEVERANCE

If cultivating these traits and keeping them in balance sounds like an overwhelming challenge--it is--unless you are selective and take one small step at a time. It takes perseverance to keep them in perspective. The following can help you in achieving balance:

Independence / Dependence

Keeping your illness in perspective means not letting it become your total preoccupation--not allowing yourself to become your illness. This can lead to over-dependence and unnecessary limitation. On the other hand, going to extremes of independence based on an unrealistic under-estimation of the seriousness of

189

your impairment can do harm in the other direction. For example, denial can lead to the under-use of sound strategies of intervention and helpful supports. An appropriate balance and goal is mature interdependence.

Acceptance / Constructive Rebellion

An example of attitudes which seem paradoxical is the fact that you are told to accept your illness, but also told to fight. This can be confusing. How much should your acceptance encompass? It is important to accept the reality of your illness, and to accept your body with all its limitations. Although this can be difficult, it is possible, as demonstrated by Alice Walker when she wrote, "...and I saw that it was possible to love it (her damaged eye); that, in fact, for all it had taught me, of shame and anger and inner vision, I <u>did</u> love it."[2]

But it's not necessary or wise to accept the limitations that are imposed by man's inhumanity to man. Sonda Aronson knows better than to accept distorted attitudes toward disabled artists. She and Neil Marcus both demonstrate courageous non-acceptance and constructive fighting when they take action for more access for the physically impaired.

It's also important to understand the difference between acceptance and resignation. Resignation is a giving up and a wiping out of self. Acceptance is an assertive act of the will, a saying "yes" to the inevitable, a voluntary acceptance of the obligatory. It is the decision to stop beating your head against a stone wall and to save that energy for more rewarding efforts.

Solitude / Sociability

Often our respondents spoke of the need to spend time alone, especially when they are in pain. There is a need for time for contemplation whether that takes the form of prayer, meditation or just rest. Dag Hammarskjold, former Secretary-General of the United Nations, wrote in *Markings*:

> *The Longest Journey*
> *Is the journey inwards*
> *Of him who has chosen his destiny.*

To do an adequate job of self-assessment, to develop insight, and to come to decisions about how you plan to respond to the changes in your life, requires time alone.

There is a pitfall in too much isolation, however, as it can feed depression. Everyone needs people. As a Unitarian Minister, Anthony Perrino said, "When the world comes crashing down, and we sit among the ruins of yesterday's hopes, dreams, and blithe assumptions, it is love alone that can give us the strength to face another day; the fact is that this fragile fabric we call humanity is held together by the gossamer threads of human affection."

Seriousness / Humor

To say that humor should not be taken lightly may sound like a contradiction in terms, but humor is important in serious ways to everyone, especially to those who are ill. Laughter, sometimes called inner jogging, lowers levels of tension, and tension can exacerbate physical as well as emotional symptoms. Henry Ward Beecher wrote that:

> *A person without a sense of humor is like a wagon without*
> *springs, jolted by every pebble in the road.*

The Old Testament has something to say about the significance of humor in relation to illness:

> *A merry heart doeth like a good medicine.*

> The Book of Proverbs

The importance of humor and positive attitudes have become more and more recognized. Norman Cousins'[3] approach to his illness, which included his renting old Marx Brothers films as part of his cure, is not only often quoted, but also has gained wide respect. However, humor that is at the expense of another person is not healing humor. Humor that helps people see and enjoy the ridiculousness of situations is healthy, is "ice-breaking," and is a high level of communication. But it is more than that. It serves the sense of wholeness. If you can laugh at yourself in ludicrous circumstances, you are reflecting and reinforcing your sense of transcendence, your identity apart from the event. And transcendence is the goal.

But everyone wants to be taken seriously some of the time. The person who feels that life is not more than a barrel of laughs comes across as clownish and shallow. You want to keep developing your sense of humor, but surely not at the expense of the serious side of your nature.

Purposefulness / Flexibility

Victor Frankl, while in a concentration camp, wondered why some prisoners survived, and some did not, apart from any measures of physical strength or constitutional factors. He believed that the difference was a sense of purpose. It's interesting to speculate that perhaps the purpose in life is to find a purpose in life. Every one of our profiled transcenders has been forced to give up some previously held life goals, and several of them, as well as many of the people who responded to questionnaires, reported that this shift is from materialistic to more intellectual or spiritual goals. Many reported that an interest in higher education and/or careers would never have been developed had it not been for their illness.

A sense of purpose provides a criteria for evaluating opportunities. Seed catalogues are intriguing if you are planning a garden. Dry medical tomes suddenly become relevant if your goal is to find out more about your disease. When you decide you want to learn a new skill, certain articles, television programs, or people can suddenly attract your enthusiastic attention where previously they would have gone ignored. Your purpose may be purely practical, such as learning to brush your teeth with impaired arms; it may be political, like participating in demonstrations with A.D.A.P.T. (Americans Disabled for Accessible Public Transportation); or it may be spiritual if you believe, as Guy Murchie expressed in *The Seven Mysteries of Life*, that God may have created us to develop spirit. Your purpose may be to rid the world of hunger, to help families cope with chronic illness by providing counseling, to change public attitudes through art or drama, or to contribute to public knowledge through computer science or astronomy. May Sarton writes in *Journal of a Solitude*[4] that, "It is only when we can believe that we are creating the soul that life has any meaning, but when we can believe it--and I do and always have--then there is nothing we do that is without meaning and nothing that we suffer that does not hold the seed of creation in it." So to nurture that seed of creativity it is important to develop a sense of purpose.

But your purpose must not be rigid. Initially it takes great flexibility to make the necessary shifts in your goals, and even after that, unless flexibility is maintained, imbalances will occur. Rigid personalities have a much harder time making adjustments to changes in their lives, especially the devastating changes that chronic illness brings.

Planfulness / Spontaneity

Once you have a sense of purpose and have set some goals, your plan becomes your way of implementing them. The art lies in designing your plan so that the activities are never beyond your abilities. Your plan should also incorporate built-in rewards, and be loosely enough structured so that there are allowances for breaks, for play, for spontaneous reactions to the unexpected--for fun.

Amye Leong develops masterful plans to realize her goals, but she remains "young at heart." Abbie Spellman swims to raise funds to end world hunger, but she also swims for fun. With all its pain and all the careful scheduling for doctor, hospital, and other therapy appointments, the lives of Ken and Maggie are full of music and playfulness. Jeanne Naspo and Joyce Kisheneff work hard at their professions, but they still take time out to relax with their families or go shopping. In short the profiled role models seem to have achieved a balance between planfulness and spontaneity, purposeful work and spontaneous play.

Self-Care / Concern for Others

Stewardesses on airplanes are careful to warn passengers to place the oxygen mask over their own face before placing one over their child's face. The rationale is that you are not much good to your child if you are dead. Unless many of your basic needs are met, you are not in a position to extend much help to others. You need to be your own best friend in order to be a good friend to others; to be gentle with yourself--not judge yourself too harshly--so that you'll know how to be gentle and not too judgmental toward others. Nancy Mairs writes in the Chapter entitled, "On Being A Cripple," in *With Wings:*[5]

> *This gentleness is part of the reason I'm not sorry I'm a cripple....It has opened and enriched my life enormously, this sense that my frailty and need must be mirrored in others, that in searching for and shaping a stable core in a life wrenched by change and loss, change and loss, I must recognize the same process, under individual conditions, in the lives around me. I do not deprecate such knowledge, however I've come by it.*

Empathy for others is often born out of suffering, and lays the basis for the kind of equilibrium that brings self-care and care for others into viable balance

Positive self-Image / Positive Image of Others

Self-concepts are by definition, subjective and often irrational as well. For example, emaciated anorexics see themselves as fat, many old people see themselves as youthful, and some thirty-year olds see themselves as old and wrinkled. The goal is not objectivity, or even rationality, but self-knowledge about your specific needs. From this can emerge the self-care skills that help you meet those needs and make you feel better about yourself.

To Doris who had cancer, losing her hair was more difficult than losing her breasts, so wigs had more priority than prosthetic bras. Self-knowledge also engenders healthy, realistic self-esteem. When some people see Neil Marcus they may see a twisted body, a frame in "dystonic disarray." But Neil, the successful playwright/actor/poet/humorist, sees himself as a "fantastic spastic mime creatively endowed with disability." Giving yourself credit where it is due, focusing on what you find acceptable in yourself, eventually gets you past the self-centeredness (regression) that illness brings, to a stronger and more positive sense of self. Then you can see beyond your own needs to the concerns of others. It is a question of attitude and an attitude is simply an accumulation of habitual patterns of thought:

> *Your mind will be like its habitual thoughts; for the soul becomes dyed with the color of its thoughts.*

> Marcus Aurelius

The fact that wholeness in the sense of self can come out of chronically ill bodies was evident in statements of transcenders. "I've developed a greater tolerance of my imperfections and those of others. I've developed patience, positive thinking, and greater spirituality," said one. "I've learned not to judge people so quickly," said another. "I have greater empathy for others and animals; I have a stronger sense of who I am," wrote still another.

Faith and Trust / Healthy Skepticism

Faith is a confident belief in the truth, value, or trustworthiness of a person, idea, or thing without logical proof or material evidence. It is a powerful option. Amye Leong describes her faith as a belief in a positive outcome, while Elsa Campbell believes that love, as described in I Corinthians, is what life is all about.

195

Experts now suspect that a belief system can translate expectation into actual physiological change. That belief can be faith in the inner strength that is in all of us, that mainspring of life that leads us to grow toward the light, just as plants do.

But how disastrous it is if your faith is the naively blind sort that influences you to believe in con operations that exploit the sick, or spend great amounts of money on fraudulent "cures." A balance between faith and skepticism is important for survival.

Toughness / Accommodation

To paraphrase Art Linkletter's title, *Aging Is Not For Sissies*, chronic illness is not for sissies, either. It takes a certain toughness, as you well know. But there is irony in how this toughness gets balanced with a capacity for accommodation. Gretal Erlich in *The Solace of Open Spaces*[6] writes, "The toughness I was learning was not martyred doggedness, a dumb heroism, but the art of accommodation. I thought: to be tough is to be fragile; to be tender is to be truly fierce."

Abbie Spellman exhibits both sides of this paradox when she swims with fierce determination, but is gently accommodating with the handicapped children who are her swimming buddies. This combination of toughness and tenderness can be identified in several of the transcenders, and perhaps you can recognize it in yourself.

There are many other traits that translate into a question of balance. Erlich also juxtaposes loss with gain when she writes, "The lessons of impermanence taught me this: loss constitutes an odd kind of fullness; despair empties out into an unquenchable appetite for life."

The task is to keep a kind of dynamic balance between these opposing tendencies, an equilibrium between extremes. It is a difficult task because it's easy to over-correct, and thus fall into another distorted, one-sided position. Brian Stonehill, in a review of Anthony Storr's book *Solitude: A Return to Self* (L.A. Times 'Book Review,' August 28, 1988) wrote, "I like to think of a ladder:

one foot to the left of your center of gravity, and one foot to the right, and so on and up we go. It's easy to miss the ladder's edge between correction and over compensation."

Of course, imbalances will occur almost daily. The trait that is the underpinning, the lynch-pin that holds all the other traits together in a workable balance, and gets you back on track, is perseverance. With perspective and perseverance you can cultivate the traits you select, keep them in balance, and advance toward transcendence. Probably one of the best examples of someone who has transcended his illness and balanced his life is Stephen Hawking whose profile follows.

Stephen Hawking: Explorer of the Universe

Dr. Stephen William Hawking is a professor of mathematics at Cambridge University, and is widely regarded as the greatest theoretical physicist since Albert Einstein. Suffering from Amyotrophic lateral sclerosis, ALS (known as Lou Gehrig's Disease) he is still a giant in the field of astronomy. His goal in his words is, "a complete understanding of the universe - why it is as it is and why it exists at all." He is making progress toward that goal, advancing beyond Einstein's theory of relativity to the subatomic world of quantum mechanics, where elementary particles behave unpredictably. He is best known for his calculations of the physics of the hypothetical apertures in the fabric of space-time known as black holes.

In the 1984 *Current Biography Yearbook,* it is stated that Hawking's ability to soar creatively in cosmological thought has been "abetted" by a severe physical disability. He is suffering from what has been called his 26-year losing battle with ALS. A close colleague, Roger Penrose, believes that Hawking's condition has forced him to work more creatively, to take imaginative leaps where someone with a less uncertain future might want to cogitate a little longer. Hawking himself dismisses that notion utterly. The only effect of ALS on his work that he is willing to concede is that "I avoid problems with a lot of equations, because

I cannot manage to do them in my head. But,"he adds, "those are the most boring problems."

Along with the brilliance of his mind, his courage is legendary. His early symptoms were slurred speech, and difficulty in tying his shoes. In 1963 he was struck by the slow, wasting neuromuscular disorder of ALS, for which there is no known cure. It involves deterioration of the motor neurons of the spinal cord, medulla, and cortex. It disables skeletal muscles, affecting speech, swallowing, limbs, and shoulders and usually ending in fatal atrophy of the chest muscles. On the bright side, if it may be called that, it is, according to its victims, painless, and fortunately for a thinker such as Hawking, it does not affect the brain or the senses.

Before receiving his B.A. degree at Oxford, in 1962, Hawking considered staying on at that university for graduate work in astronomy, but the observatory there was equipped only for the observation of sunspots, and he was more interested in theory than in observation. He decided to go to Cambridge where they did work on theoretical astronomy and cosmology which applies creative thinking as well as scientific knowledge to the study of the character of the universe. He is quoted as saying that he found cosmology, "exciting because it really did seem to involve the big question: Where did the universe come from?"

It was right after he started at Cambridge that his symptoms developed. The depression that resulted prevented him from making much progress in research. After about two years his disease began to stabilize, and when he realized that he would survive, albeit disabled, his natural buoyancy returned. His mentor, Dennis W. Sciama, encouraged him to get back to work on his Ph.D.

Hawking identifies the real turning point as his marriage to Jane Wilde, a student of languages, in 1965. John Boslough in *Science* (November, 1981), quotes Hawking on his marriage, "It made me determined to live...and it was about that time that I began making professional progress." Now they have three children, two boys and a girl, the youngest born in 1979. Despite his disease and the distractions and pressures that go with being a celebrity, he and his wife have managed to maintain a decent, happy, balanced family life.

Hawking and his friend and collaborator, Roger Penrose, applied a new and intricate mathematical method of their own devising to the general theory of relativity, developed by Albert Einstein to explain how gravity affects the behavior of the universe and its large systems. Hawking's book, *A Brief History of Time: From the Big Bang to Black Holes*, (Bantam Books) remained on the New York Times Best Seller list for over six months, which may seem surprising because of its erudition, but it makes fundamental questions of the universe accessible.

Stephen Hawking cannot walk; he uses a motorized wheelchair which he steers with a joy stick. He cannot feed himself; his meals are fed to him by a nurse. He cannot talk; his computers are cleverly designed for someone who can make only one movement. The cursor flicks among the letters of the alphabet, stopping at one when he squeezes his switch; this calls up a screen full of pre-programmed words beginning with the chosen letter. After Hawking chooses a word, it is added to a sentence at the bottom of the screen ready to be pronounced in a metallic voice from a speaker behind his seat. Dr. Hawking's mind transcends all of these constraints and goes soaring on to the galaxies to increase man's knowledge of the universe.

STEPS YOU CAN TAKE TO DEVELOP TRAITS TO HELP YOU SOAR

- Refer back to the Balanced Traits Chart at the beginning of this Chapter and assess where you are in relation to the traits that have been discussed. Select which ones you want to develop further

- Search for people, historical and contemporary, who have the same illness that you have. Select one for a role model. Find out about his or her personality traits and how he or she has developed them.

- Identify an area where you could be nicer to yourself, and a situation where you could show more concern for others. Plan to take action in both.

CONCLUSION

Living creatively with a chronic illness requires skills and support to transcend the losses, pain, and frustrations. First you feel like a victim, grieving losses. Then, as you develop skills, and identify the turning points in your growth, you will develop parts of your personality that would have remained dormant had it not been for your illness and your efforts to transcend.

You can spiral upward inwardly and spiritually regardless of what is happening to your body. That is what transcendence is all about.

NOTES

APPENDIX

Appendix

SUGGESTED READINGS

Alberti, Robert E. and Emmons, Michael L., *Your Perfect Right: a Guide to Assertive Living* (Fifth Edition), Impact Publishers, Inc., San Luis Obispo, CA, 5th ed. 1986

Augsburger, David, *Caring Enough to Forgive/Not to Forgive*, Regal Books, Ventura, CA, 1981

Berne, Eric, *Beyond Games And Scripts*, Grove Press, New York, l976

Biermann, June and Tohey, Barbara, *The Diabetic's Total Health Book*, Tarcher, Los Angeles, 1982

Borysenko, Joan, Ph.D., *Minding The Body, Mending The Mind*, Bantam Books, New York. 1987

Buscaglia, Leo F., *Personhood*, Fawcett Columbine, New York, 1978

Burns, David, M.D., *Feeling Good: The New Mood Therapy*, Signet, New York, 1980

Carroll, Thomas J., *Blindness: What It Is, What It Does, And How To Live With It*, Little Brown and Company, l961

Chester, Laura, *Lupus Novice: Toward Self-healing*, Station Hill Press, Inc., Barrytown, NY 12507, 1987

Colgrove, Melba, Bloomfield, and McWilliams, Peter, *How To Survive The Loss Of A Love*, Bantam Books, Inc. New York, 1976

Cousins, Norman, *Anatomy Of An Illness; As Perceived By The Patient; Reflections On Healing And Regeneration*, W.W. Norton, New York 1979

Cousins, Norman, *The Healing Heart*, W. W. Norton, New York, 1983

Edelwich, Jerry, and Brodsky, Archie, *Diabetes: Caring For Your Emotions As Well As Your Health*, Addison-Wesley pub. Co., Inc. New York, 1986

Ellis, Albert A., and Harper R., *A New Guide To Rational Living*, Wilshire Books, Hollywood, CA 1979

Elgin, Suzette H. *The Gentle Art Of Verbal Self-defense*, Harper and Row, New York, 1986

Erlich, Gretel, *The Solace Of Open Spaces*, Penguin Books Inc. New York, 1986

Frankl, Victor, *Man's Search For Meaning*, Simon and Schuster, New York, 3rd Ed. 1984

Heller, Joseph and Vogel, Speed, *No Laughing Matter*, Avon Books, New York,1986

Heiss, Gayle, *Living Well With Chronic Illness*, Q.E.D. Press, Fort Bragg, CA, 1987

Jampolsky, Jerry, with Hopkins, Patricia and Thetford William N., *Teach Only Love: Seven Principles Of Attitudinal Healing*, Bantam Books, New York, 1983

Jovanovic, Lois, M.D., Biermann, June, and Barbara Toohey, *The Diabetic Woman*, Jeremy P. Tarcher, Inc, L. A. 1987

Keirsey, David and Bates, Marilyn, *Please Understand Me: Character And Temperament Types*, Prometheus Nemesis Books, Del Mar, CA, 1978

Knight, Bob, *Psychotherapy With Older Adults*, Sage Publications, Inc. Beverly Hills, CA, 1986

LeMaistre, JoAnn, *Beyond Rage: The Emotional Impact Of Chronic Physical Illness*, Alpine Guild, Oak Park, IL, 1988

Lewis, Kathleen S., *Successful Living With Chronic Illness*, Avery Publishing Group, Inc., New Jersey, 1985

Lindbergh, Ann Morrow, *Hour Of Lead: Sharing Sorrow*, Redpath Press

Lord, Janice Harris, *Beyond Sympathy: What To Say or Do For Someone Suffering an Injury, Illness, or Loss*, Pathfinder Publishing, 458 Dorothy Ave., Ventura, CA 93003, 1989

Mairs, Nancy, *Plain Text: Essays By Nancy Mairs* (a multiple sclerosis survivor) University of Arizona Press, Tucson, Arizona, 1986

McCoy, Doris Lee, *Megatraits: 12 Traits Of Successful People*, Wordware Publishing, Inc., Plano, Texas, 1988

Murchie, Guy, *The Seven Mysteries Of Life,* Houghton Mifflin Co., 1978

Phillips,. Robert H., Ph.D., *Coping With Lupus,* Avery Publishing Group, Inc., New Jersey, 1984

Pitzele, Sefra dKobrin, *We Are Not Alone: Learning To Live With A Chronic Illness*, Workman Publishing, New York 1987

Pitzele, Sefra Kobrin, One More Day: *Daily Meditations for People with Chronic Illness*, Harper & Row, New York, 1988.

Progoff, Ira, *The Intensive Journal* and *At A Journal Workshop: The Basic Text And Guide For Using The Intensive Journal*, Dialogue House Library, New York, 1975

Register, Cheri, *Living With Chronic Illness: Days Of Patience And Passion*, Free Press, New York, 1987

Resnick, Rose, *Dare To Dream: The Rose Resnick Story*,Strawberry Hill Press, San Francisco, 1988

Rosner, Louis J., Ph.D. and Ross, Shelley, *Multiple Sclerosis: New Hope and Practical Gudelines For People With M.S. And Their Families*, Prentice Hall Press, 1987

Rubin, Theodore Isaac, *Compassion And Self-hate: An Alternative To Despair*, Ballantine, New York 1975

Sarton, May, *Journal Of A Solitude*, W.W. Norton and Co., New York, 1973

Siegel, Bernard S. M.D. *Love, Medicine And Miracles*, Harper and Row, New York, 1986

Simonton, Stephanie Matthews, *The Healing Family*, Bantam Books, New York, 1984

Stoddard, Alexandra, *Living A Beautiful Life*, Random House, New York, 1986

Strong, Maggie, *Mainstay: For The Well Spouse Of The Chronically Ill: A Moving Personal Account And A Companion Guide*, Little, Brown & Co., Boston, 1988

Tournier, Paul, *Learn To Grow Old*, Harper and Row, 10. E. 53rd St., New York 10022 1983

Viorst, Judith, *Necessary Losses: The Loves, Illusions, Dependencies, And Impossible Expectations That All Of Us Have To Give Up In Order To Grow*, Simon and Schuster, New York, 1986

With Wings, Eds: Saxton, Marsha and Howe, Florence. The Feminist Press, New York, 1987

RESOURCES

American Heart Association
7320 Greenville Ave.
Dallas, TX 75231

Arthritis Foundation
1314 Spring St., N.W.
Atlanta, GA 30309
(404) 872-7100

The Arthritis Society
920 Yonge Street, Suite 240
Toronto M4Y 357
Ontario, Canada

National Institute Of Arthritis,
Musculoskeletal And Skin Diseases
9000 Rockville Pike
Bethesda, MD 20892
(301) 496-3583

Better Breathers
Contact local lung association for support group.

American Cancer Society
4 West 35th St.
New York, NY 10001
(212) 736-3030

National Cancer Institute
9000 Rockville Pike
Bethesda, MD 20892

Chronic Fatigue Immune Dysfunction Syndrome (CFIDS) Society
P.O. Box 230108
Portland, Oregon 97223

Appendix

Federal Centers For Disease Control
1600 Clifton Rd. NE
Building 6, Room 127
Atlanta, GA 30333
(404) 329-3091

American Diabetes Association
1660 Duke St.
Alexandria, VA 22313
(703) 549-1500

National Institute Of Diabetes,
Kidney And Digestive Diseases
9000 Rockville Pike
Bethesda, MD 20892
(301) 496-3583

Disabled Artists' Network
P.O. Box 20781
New York, NY 10025 (Include a stamped self-addressed envelope)

American Heart Association
7320 Greenville Ave.
Dallas, TX 75231
(214) 750-5300

National Heart, Lung, And
Blood Institute
7550 Wisconsin Ave.
Bethesda, MD 20892
(301) 496-4868

Independent Living For The Disabled Office, Hud
7th and D. Streets, SW
Washington, DC 20410

Intersticial Cystitis Association Of America (West Coast)
P.O. Box 151323
San Diego, CA 92115

Intersticial Cystitis Association Of America (East Coast)
P.O. Box 1553,
Madison Square Station
New York, N.Y.10159

Kidney, Urologic, And Hematological Diseases
5333 Westward Ave.
Bethesda, MD 20892
(301) 496-7458

Leukemia Society Of America, Inc.
733 Third Ave.
New York, NY 10017
(212) 573-8484

American Lung Association
1740 Broadway
New York, NY 10019
(212) 315-8700

Lupus Foundation Of America, Inc.
1717 Massachusetts Ave., N.W. Suite 203
Washington, DC 20036
(800) 558-0121

National Lupus Erythematosus Foundation
5430 Van Nuys Boulevard, Suite 206
Van Nuys, CA 91401
(818) 885-8787

Mended Hearts
Contact local heart association for support groups.

Myasthenia Gravis Foundation
7-11 S. Broadway
White Plains, NY 10601
(914) 328-1717

Appendix

National Easter Seal Society For Crippled
Children And Adults
2023 West Ogden Ave.
Chicago, IL 60612

National Digestive Diseases Educational
Information Clearing House
1255 23rd St., N.W.
Washington, D.C. 20037
(202) 296-1138

National Information Center For The Handicapped
P.O. Box 1492
Washington, DC 20013

National Multiple Sclerosis Society
205 East 42nd St.
New York, NY 10017
(212) 986-3240

National Neurofibromatosis Foundation
141 Fifth Avenue, Suite 7-s
New York, NY 10010

National Association For The Visually
Handicapped
305 East 24th Street, 17-c
New York, NY 10010

National Clearing House For Human Genetic Diseases
805 15th Street, N.W., Suite 500
Washington, DC 20005
(202) 842-7617

National Kidney Foundation, Inc
2 Park Ave.
New York, NY 10016
(212) 889-2210

National Institute Of Neurological And
Communication Disorders And Stroke
9000 Rockville Pike
Bethesda, MD 20892 (301) 496-5751

National Organization Of Rare Disorders
P.O. Box 8923
New Fair Field, CT 06812

Parkinson's Disease Foundation
Columbia Presbyterian Medical Center
650 West 168th St.
New York, NW 10032
(212) 923-4700

People-to-People Committee For The Handicapped
1028 Connecticut Avenue, NW
Washington, DC 20036

Polio Information Center
610 Main Street, Suite A446
Roosevelt Island, NY 10046

International Polio Network
Gazette International Networking Institute
4502 Maryland Ave.
St. Louis, MO 63108
(314) 361-0475

Retinitis Pigmentosa - International
P. O. Box 900
Woodland Hills, CA 91365

Siblings Information Network
Department of Health & Human Services
Room #340 E. Humphrey Building
Washington, DC 20201

Appendix

Stroke Club International
805 12th St.
Galveston, TX 77550
(403) 762-1022

Sugar Free Center
P.O. Box 114
Van Nuys, CA 91408
(818) 994-1093

GLOSSARY

Amyotrophic Lateral Sclerosis (Lou Gehrig's Disease): A motor neuron disease characterized by progressive degeneration of the nervous system so that both voluntary and involuntary muscle control is lost.

Ankylosing Spondylitis: A form of arthritis that causes inflammation of the joints of the spine, so that bones fuse, or grow together.

Arthritis: Joint inflammation; refers to more than 100 different diseases.

Autoimmune disorder: A condition in which the body malfunctions and attacks itself by making antibodies against its own cells, causing tissue injury and inflammation.

Chronic fatigue syndrome: A cluster of symptoms often including exhaustion, difficulty concentrating, headache, sore throat, muscle pains, fevers, and tender lymph glands, and of probable multiple causes including a malfunctioning immune system.

Chronic illness: A disease which lasts for many years; perhaps for a lifetime.

Circulatory system: Of or pertaining to the system of the body that produces the blood/oxygen supply.

Connective tissue: The tissue that binds the body together, such as cartilage, muscles, tendons, ligaments, and skin.

Diabetes: A disorder of the metabolic system that affects how the body uses food, causing sugar levels to be too high. The major types are Type I (insulin production by the pancreas is ineffective), and Type II (body is unable to use the insulin it makes).

Diabetic retinopathy: A disease of the eye concerning the retina, the membrane at the back of the inside of the eyeball which receives light and images.

Dystonia: A rare neurological disorder that affects the coordination of muscles, and the transmission of messages from brain to muscles.

Ego: The self; the person we perceive ourselves to be.

Ego states: Parts of the self that are dynamic and observable.

Endometriosis: Chronic inflammation of the endrometrium, or the inner mucous membrane of the uterus.

Endorphins: A hormone similar to morphine which is produced by the body as a natural pain control substance.

Epstein-Barr virus (EPV): A virus of the herpes group, with fevers, extreme fatigue, and flu-like symptoms. Can become chronic.

Fibromyalgia: A rheumatic condition that causes inflammation, pain, and stiffness in the connective tissue around the joints.

Fight/Flight anxiety response: A mental and physical state in which the body/mind prepares for action; to either fight or flee. Pupils dilate, blood pressure rises, muscles contract, adrenalin flows, etc.

Friedrich's ataxia: A slowly progressive disorder of the muscles and nervous system causing an inability to coordinate voluntary muscle movements.

Gout: A form of arthritis in which the body builds up excess uric acid; uric acid crystals collect in the joints causing pain.

Guillian-Barre: An acute usually rapidly progressive form of polyneuropathy. Characterized by muscular weakness and mild distal sensory loss that about half the time begins five days to three weeks after surgery, or an immunization

Hunger Project: A global effort to end hunger on the planet by year 2000.

Immune system: The body's natural defense system against injury and infection.

Juvenile rheumatoid arthritis: A general term that refers to several kinds of arthritis that occur in children.

Metabolism: The physical and chemical changes that occur in the body as food is broken down and used to provide energy necessary for maintenance and growth.

Multiple sclerosis: A degenerative disease of the central nervous system in which there is a hardening of tissue in the brain and/or spinal cord. This interferes with the brain's ability to control functions.

Muscular dystrophy: A group of related diseases in which there is progressive wasting of muscles; origin is unknown.

Myofascial pain syndrome: Migratory pain that continues beyond the time of healing from an injury of soft tissue.

Nervous system: All the nerve cells and nervous tissue in an organism that coordinates and controls movement.

Osteoarthritis: The most common form of arthritis, it involves the breakdown of cartilage and other joint tissues, so that bone rubs against bone.

Parkinson's disease: A disorder of the nervous system characterized by rhythmic tremors and muscle rigidity, creating slowness of movement.

Poliomyelitis: An acute infectious disease caused by a viral inflammation in the spinal cord, producing paralysis, muscle atrophy, often with permanent deformity.

Post polio syndrome: A condition of worn out muscles, with attendant pain, experienced decades later by polio sufferers.

Project F.O.O.D.: Food Out Of Donations, a charitable effort to eliminate hunger at the local level (Ventura, CA) co-sponsored by Project Understanding, a non-profit ministry, and the farmers of the Ventura Certified Farments Market.

Respiratory system: The system of organs involved in the exchange of carbon dioxide and oxygen between an organism and its environment.

Retinal hemorrhage: Tiny blood vessels breaking in the retina of the eye, causing vision loss.

Retinitis Pigmentosa: A disease of the eye, in which there is slowly progressive bilateral retinal degeneration.

Rheumatic diseases: A group of diseases that attaack muscles, ligaments, tendons, joints, and sometimes other body parts.

Rheumatoid arthritis: A common systemic form of arthritis in which there is inflammation and permanent damage to the joint tissues. This is an autoimmune disease.

Sabin: Albert Sabin was a Russian born U.S. physician and bacteriologist who developed an oral vaccine to prevent poliomyelitis.

Salk: Jonas Salk is a U.S. physician and bacteriologist who developed a vaccine for injection to prevent poliomyelitis.

Syndrome: A number of symptoms occurring together and characterizing a specific disease or condition.

Systemic lupus erythematosus: An autoimmune rheumatic disease that often affects the skin, joints, and sometimes internal organs. It can also involve other connective tissue and blood cells.

END NOTES

Introduction:

1. Murchie, Guy, *The Seven Mysteries of Life: An Exploration in Science and Philosophy*, Houghton Mifflin Co., Boston, 1978.

Chapter 2:

1. Viorst, Judith, *Necessary Losses,* Simon and Schuster, New York, 1986

Chapter 3:

1. Poem by Nicholas Lentine, Whittier, CA 90605

2. Frankl, Victor, *Man's Search for Meaning*, Simon and Schuster, New York, NY, 3rd Ed., 1984.

3. Melinkoff, Ellen, *Singles Scene*, Los Angeles Times, January 26, 1987.

4. From the Health Examiner, Gold Coast Edition, March 1988. P.O. Box 4272, Saticoy, CA 93005 (Managing Eds. Burton and Marsha Danet).

5. Poem by Brett St. Giles.

Chapter 4:

1. Buscaglia, Leo F., *Personhood*, Fawcett Columbine, New York, NY, 1978.

Chapter 5:

1. Strong, Maggie, *Mainstay: For the Well Spouse of the Chronically Ill: A Moving Personal Account and a Companion Guide*, Little, Brown & Co., Boston, 1988.

Chapter 7:

1. Heller, Joseph, and Vogel, Speed, *No Laughing Matter*, Avon Books, New York, NY, 1986.

2. Alberti, Robert E. and Emmons, Michael L. *Your Perfect Right: A Guide to Assertive Living*, Impact Publishers, San Luis Obispo, CA, Fifth Edition, 1986.

3. Register, Cheri. *Living with Chronic Illness: Days of Patience and Passion*, Free Press, New York, NY, 1987.

4. Young Et Heart, Arthritis Support Group for the Young and Active, 29936 Knoll View Drive, Palos Verdes, CA 90274, Amye Leong, MBA, President and Founder.

5. Elgin, Suzette Haden, *The Gentle Art of Verbal Self Defense*, Prentice Hall, New York, NY 10023, 1986

Chapter 8:

1. Butler, Robert, Former Director of the National Counsel on Aging and author of Aging and Mental Health and Why Survive: Being Old in America.

2. Progoff, Ira, *At a Journal Workshop*, Dialogue House Library, 45 West 10th ST., New York, NY 10011, 1975.

3. Tournier, Paul, *Learn To Grow Old*, Harper and Row, 10 E. 53rd St. New York, NY 10022.

4. Lord, Janice Harris, *No Time for Goodbyes*, Pathfinder Publishing, Ventura CA, 1988.

5. Campbell, Elsa K., *Healing the Trauma of Diabetic Vision Loss*, Unpublished thesis submitted in partial fulfillment of the requirements for the degree of "Master of Arts in Counseling Psychology," Human Relations Institute, Santa Barbara, CA, 1987.

Chapter 9:

1. Peterson, Charles M. MD, and Jovanovic, Lois, MD., *The Diabetes Self-Care Method*, Simon and Schuster, Inc. NY (A Fireside Book), 1979, 1984. A married couple, she with diabetes, he Director of Research at the Sansum Medical Foundation, Santa Barbara, CA.

Chapter 10.

1. Disabled Artist's Newwork, P.O. Box 20781, New York, NY 10025.

Chapter 11:

1. Colgrove, Ph.D., Bloomfield MD, and Mc. Williams, Peter. *How To Survive The Loss Of A Love*, Prelude Press (formerly Leo Press), Allen Park, MI 48101, 1976.

2. Rubin, Theodore Isaac, MD. *Compassion and Self-Hate: An Alternative to Despair*, Ballantine Books, New York, NY, 1975.

3. Stoddard, Alexandra. *Living A Beautiful Life: 500 Ways To Add Elegance, Order, Beauty and Joy to Every Day of Your Life*, Random House, New York, NY, 1986.

Chapter 12:

1. Song written by Sharon Riddell of Artistry Productions, P.O. Box 158056, Nashville, TN 37215.

2. Ellis, Albert A., & Harper, R. *A New Guide to Rational Living*, Wilshire Books, Hollywood, CA 1979.

3. Berne, Eric, *Beyond Games and Scripts*, Grove Press, New York, NY 1976.

Chapter 13:

1. Chester, Laura, *Lupus Novice*, Station Hill Press, Inc., Barrytown, NY 12507, 1987.

Chapter 14:

1. Excerpt from *Love, Medicine and Miracles* by Bernie S. Siegel, MD. Copyright 1986 by Bernie S. Siegel, S. Korman, and A. Schiff, Trustees of the Bernard S. Siegel Childrens Trust Fund. Reprinted by permission of Harper & Row, Publishers, Inc.

2. With Wings: *An Anthology of Literature By and About Women with Disabilities*, Eds: Marsha Saxton and Florence Howe, The Feminist Press at The City University of New York, NY 1987.

3. Cousins, Norman. *Anatomy of an Illness; As Perceived by the Patient; Reflections on Healing and Regeneration*, W.W. Norton, New York, NY 1979.

4. Sarton, May. *Journal of A Solitude*, W.W.Norton and Co., New York, NY, 1973.

5. Mairs, Nancy, On Being A Cripple. From *With Wings*: *An Anthology of Literature By and About Women with Disabilities*, Eds: Marsha Saxton and Florence Howe, The Feminist Press at The City University of New York, NY 1987

6. Erlich, Gretel. *The Solace of Open Spaces*, Penguin Books Inc. New York, NY 1986.

INDEX

ORDER FORM

Pathfinder Publishing
458 Dorothy Ave.
Ventura, CA 93003
Telephone (805)642-9278

Please send me the following books from Pathfinder Publishing:

___Copies of **Beyond Sympathy**@$9.95.........................$_____

___Copies of **Living Creatively With Chronic Illness**
@$11.95 ....$_____

___Copies of **No Time For Goodbyes** @ $8.95.............$_____

___Copies of **Quest For Respect** @ 6.95 ....$_____

___Copies of **Stop Justice Abuse** @ $10.95 each...........$_____

Sub-Total...$_____

Californians: Please add 6% tax. ....$_____

Shipping & Handling ....$_____

Grand Total ....$_____

I understand that I may return the book for a full refund if not satisfied.

Name:_____

Organization:_____

Address:_____

_____

ZIP:_____

Shipping: $1.75 for the first book and .50c for each additional book.